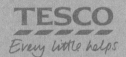

KT-166-009

Glycaemic Index
tested

the
Gi GUIDE

Understanding the Glycaemic Index,
healthy eating, lifestyle and shopping
for you and your family

Rick Gallop & Tesco

While we have taken every care to ensure that the information contained in this book is accurate and up to date, neither Tesco nor Virgin Books nor the authors accept any responsibility for illness or injury caused as a result of advice given. Please consult your doctor prior to starting any diet or activity plan. Availability of Tesco food products will vary from store to store and all references were correct at the time of going to press.

Useful links
www.britishcycling.org.uk
www.dh.gov.uk
www.diabetes.org.uk
www.gidiet.com
www.nutricentre.com
www.raceforlife.org
www.runnersworld.co.uk
www.tescodiets.com
www.tesco.com/health
www.tesco.com/healthyliving
www.tesco.com/sport

This edition published in Great Britain in 2006 by

Virgin Books
Thames Wharf Studios
Rainville Road
London W6 9HA

Copyright © 2006 Green Light Foods Inc. & Tesco Stores Ltd.

The right of Rick Gallop to be identified as the author of this work has been asserted by him in accordance with the Copyright, Designs and Patents Act 1988.

This edition features a number of changes to the previous edition. The co-author of the previous edition, Hamish Renton, has not produced or consented to these changes. This book is sold subject to the condition that it shall not, by way of trade or otherwise, be lent, resold, hired out or otherwise circulated without the publisher's prior written consent in any form of binding or cover other than that in which it is published and without a similar condition including this condition being imposed upon the subsequent purchaser.

A catalogue record for the book is available from the British Library

ISBN 0 7535 1176 2

Designed by Oh Paxton, London
Printed and bound in the UK

Contents

Foreword by Sir Steve Redgrave CBE

Although I have spent years of hard training and have learned how to eat a sensible and nutritious diet, I have been really encouraged to find out more about the Glycemic Index and am very impressed by the work undertaken by Tesco in this area of food information. I am therefore very supportive of Rick and Tesco in their efforts to bring GI into the mainstream in a way that is simple and makes sense. Having had the chance to read this book I am delighted that the authors have presented GI in such an accessible way and feel sure that by following the principles in these pages you and your family can improve your health and your waistline.

Although a seasoned Olympian and endurance athlete, I had to rethink significantly how and what I was eating when I developed diabetes some years ago. Adopting the GI plan is positive and beneficial not only to those who control their diet for healthier living, but also to anyone at risk of developing the disease. I respect the condition but it does not rule my life, and initiatives like the GI plan make this so much easier. This book shows that GI is for everyone, not just those who are at risk of diabetes and other life-changing disorders such as heart disease, or those in need of shedding some weight, but for all of us who would like to be healthy and stay healthy.

Introduction

You may be under the impression that the concept of GI is only for weight loss, but the GI way of eating, with its emphasis on fruits, vegetables, whole grains, nuts, lean meat and fish and low-fat dairy, is ideal for building and nourishing young and old alike. So it's not just about weight loss – it's suitable for all the family.

We'll be explaining more about how GI works later in this book. But the basic principles are that GI is about eating 'good' carbohydrates – that is, those which are high in fibre and low in refined carbohydrates like sugar. Lower GI foods, which you will learn more about later, are digested more slowly than high GI foods, so you should concentrate on eating mainly low and medium GI foods, but you don't have to completely exclude high GI foods. Eating mainly low and medium GI foods will help to stabilise your blood sugar and energy levels, and can help you feel full for longer.

If all the family are following GI principles, this will help to establish healthy eating patterns that will live with your children throughout their adult life. This is very important to consider, especially since obesity levels in the UK are reaching epidemic proportions. One in five children in the UK is overweight and one in ten is clinically obese. More importantly and alarmingly, between 40–70 per cent of obese children will become obese adults. Although there are many different causes of obesity, including genetics, for the majority of our children, a combination of diet, environment and lifestyle is to blame.

Even if your children aren't overweight, healthy eating and an active lifestyle are always important in order to prevent bad habits later in life that could lead to them being overweight or obese, and therefore more at risk of developing diabetes, heart disease, cancer, joint problems and even depression.

Another benefit of introducing children to the GI way of eating is that it may help with attention deficit hyperactivity disorder (ADHD) or concentration difficulties. It is believed that one trigger of ADHD may be consumption of sugar*, and many children with ADHD crave high GI foods, which leads to hypoglycaemia. All high GI foods cause a rapid rise in blood sugar levels, which causes a temporary surge of energy and at the same time, hyperactivity. Soon after this energy surge comes a dip in energy, with the end result being hypoglycaemia. This will inevitably lead to irritability, poor sleeping habits and lack of concentration. In light of this, if low GI foods are eaten most of the time, especially for breakfast, blood sugar and energy levels remain stable, and this enables the child to concentrate better and stabilise their emotions.

So make sure you get all the family involved in your new GI lifestyle! To establish healthy habits and interest in nutrition, get the kids to join in when you are preparing food. Make time for the family to eat together at least two or three times a week. A recent study reported that children who regularly ate dinner with their families were more likely to have eaten at least five portions of fruits and vegetables a day. They also had fewer fried foods and soft drinks during dinner than those children who had infrequent family meals. In this book you will discover what the Glycaemic Index is all about, and how you can put it into practice.

* 'Effects of diet on behaviour and cognition in children.' Bellisle, F. *British Journal of Nutrition,* *October* 2004

1 What is the Glycaemic Index?

The Glycaemic Index (GI) is a medical term for measuring the speed at which various foods in our digestive system break down into glucose – and this is the body's source of energy. By indexing glucose at 100, all other foods are calculated against that index. So, for example, the cereal cornflakes, which digests quickly, has a Glycemic Index of 77, but porridge is calculated at 42 as it digests more slowly, and yoghurt is even lower at 14. The foods that are measured by the GI contain carbohydrates (carbs) and these are our principal source of energy.

To fully understand how GI helps you to make healthy food choices, we should take a step back and look at how carbohydrates fit into overall nutrition.

All foods fall into the following four main groups: bread, other cereals and potatoes; fruit and vegetables; milk and dairy foods; and meat, fish and alternatives. There is a fifth group of foods that contain fat and, along with foods containing sugar, these should make up the smallest part of one's diet. These groups contain varying proportions of all or some of the main nutrients, which are protein, carbohydrates and fats.

THE LOWDOWN ON FOODS

Proteins

Proteins are an essential part of your diet. One half of your body weight is made up of protein, including muscles, organs, skin and hair. Protein is required to build and repair body tissue. Proteins also slow down the digestive process, which, as we will see shortly, is key to controlling blood-sugar levels and keeping you feeling alert, full and satisfied.

As protein is found in a broad range of foods, both animal and vegetable, it is important to choose the right sort. Red meat and dairy foods, for example, are good sources of protein, but they can also be loaded with saturated fats, which we will talk more about in the next section. The best sources for protein are:

- low-fat meats trimmed of any visible fat
- skinless poultry
- seafood (not battered or breaded)
- low-fat dairy foods
- eggs
- soya-based products (e.g. Tesco Soya Milk), and even
- the humble bean (e.g. kidney beans).

Protein should be consumed at all your meals throughout the day. We tend to be protein-light at breakfast and lunch and it is not until dinner when most of us consume our main protein quotient. Protein is also a critical brain food providing essential neurotransmitters (chemical messengers) that relay messages to the brain, so you need a constant supply throughout the day to keep you alert with an active mind.

Fats

Fats are possibly the most misunderstood of the three food categories and traditionally the villain in weight control. Let's get the facts straight. Fats are absolutely essential to your diet and your digestive process. Fat does not necessarily make you fat – the amount you eat does. This is something that's difficult to control as fat tastes, well, terrific! Your body loves it because it doesn't have to waste a lot of energy in converting fat into those fat cells around your waist and hips. Your body will do everything to encourage you to eat more. Fat contains more than twice the calories of protein or carbohydrates, so the quantity we eat is critical.

It's not just how much fat we eat, it's also what type of fat we eat that can have a serious impact on our health, particularly heart problems, strokes, some major cancers, such as prostate and colon, and even Alzheimer's disease. There are four types of fat: awful, bad, good and best.

The ones to avoid are called 'hydrogenated' or 'trans' fats and these consist of vegetable oils that have been heat-treated to make them thicken at room temperature. They are frequently found in cakes, biscuits and snacks.

The other 'bad' fats are 'saturated' fats and are easily recognisable as they come from animal sources and are always solid at room temperatures, for example butter, cheese and fatty meats.

The 'good' fats are exclusively vegetable-based oils such as corn and sunflower oils, which are called 'polyunsaturated' and 'monounsaturated'. Your best choice amongst these oils are those that are highest in monounsaturated fats such as olive and rapeseed oils. These oils have a beneficial effect on cholesterol levels and are good for your heart. Olive oil is used extensively in the Mediterranean countries where they have low rates of heart disease. The two exceptions are coconut and palm oil (often called tropical oils), which may sound healthy but are in fact the only vegetable oils that are saturated fats. Because they are cheap they are found frequently in snack foods, packaged biscuits and baked goods. Try and avoid them.

While on the subject of health, especially heart health, some oils contain a wonderful substance called 'omega-3', which is found in deep-sea fish, such as salmon, as well as in flaxseed and rapeseed oils. These are the 'best' fats. Tesco offers a range of omega-3 supplements in store or online (click on 'Nutri Centre' for an even larger range of supplements).

So the two things you should remember about fats are the quantity and the type of fat. Although many of us have tried to lower our fat intake by eating leaner cuts of meat and reduced-fat milk, we

9

have also been eating more cheese and ice cream. Also, many of today's popular foods such as snacks, cereals and fast foods contain hidden fats. As a result, the total fat consumption in our diets, contrary to popular belief, has not changed significantly.

What has changed significantly is our consumption of carbohydrates, the third of our three food categories.

Carbohydrates

Carbohydrates are the main source of energy for your body and should account for 50% of your calorie intake. (Proteins typically account for 15% and fat 35% of your daily Calories, or kcals.) They are also essential for your health.

Carbohydrates are found mainly in grains, vegetables, fruits, legumes (beans and pulses) and dairy products. Your digestive system converts carbohydrates to glucose, which dissolves into your bloodstream and is transported to those parts of your body that use energy, such as your muscles and brain. Surprisingly, the brain can use up to two-thirds of the glucose in your system.

While they do contain starch and sugar, many carbohydrates are also rich in fibre, vitamins, minerals and antioxidants, all of which play a critical role in your health and help protect you from major diseases such as heart disease, stroke and cancer. This is why many nutritional and medical authorities are questioning the effects on health of some of today's popular low-carb, high-fat diets. By minimising carbohydrates you run the risk of depriving your body of many essential nutrients as indicated above. There is little gain in improving your health by losing weight while at the same time putting your health at risk with a diet that is short-changing your nutritional needs.

As with fats, it's not just how much carbohydrate we consume, it's what type of carbohydrate that is equally important. A little history is necessary here and it is a fascinating story.

HISTORY OF FOOD PROCESSING

Concurrent with the retreating glaciers of the ice age 10,000 years ago, grains (or cereals) started being cultivated for the first time. Egypt was the bread basket of the ancient world and much of its wealth came from grain production. Grain grew to become the staple food in the western world much as rice has in the eastern regions. Grains were ground by giant grinding stones propelled by air or water.

Then came the food revolution: only a couple of generations or so ago, modern high-speed steel rolling mills ground up the grain, at the same time stripping away all the fibre, oils and nutrients to form a fine white flour. This fine white flour is a basic ingredient in most of our breads, cereals, cakes and snack foods such as crackers, corn chips, pretzels and biscuits. Our grain consumption has increased by up to 50% over the last three decades.

The same revolution in food processing has had an impact on other key carbohydrates such as fruits and vegetables. About 100 years ago, most people ate food that came straight from the farm to the dinner table. With new technology all that changed. Along came prepared and processed foods. Convenience was the buzzword. Again, this has had huge effects on the nutritional and health value of the original foods. All the great food companies such as Kraft, Nestlé and Kellogg only started processing and packaging natural foods in the past century.

We now know that proteins, fats and carbohydrates make up our diets. We also know that, for nutrition and good health, it is not just the quantity of these foods we eat that matters, it's also the quality. So with this in mind, let's now look to the role that the Glycaemic Index (GI) plays in all this.

HOW DOES GI WORK FOR ME?

As we discussed at the outset, the GI measures the speed at which food breaks down in our digestive system into glucose, the body's source of energy. Here are some examples of GI ratings:

EXAMPLE OF GI RATINGS

HIGH GI		LOW GI	
FOODS	RATING	FOODS	RATING
Sugar	100	Orange	44
Baguette	95	All Bran	43
Cornflakes	84	Oatmeal	42
Rice cakes	82	Spaghetti	41
Doughnut	76	Apple	38
Bagel	72	Beans	31
Cereal bar	72	Grapefruit	25
Biscuits (plain)	69	Yogurt	14

Any food rating less than 55 in the Gi is considered low

The GI rating of a food is important to nutrition and health because:
• Low GI foods tend to have more nutritional (or healthy) content than the high GI foods, which are usually highly processed. This is important for your health.
• Low GI foods break down in your digestive system more slowly, leaving you feeling more satiated for a longer period of time so you don't go hungry. This is critical for weight control.
• Low GI foods are important for managing diseases, such as diabetes, where controlling blood-sugar levels is essential.
Let's deal with each of these in turn.

Nutrition

You can easily see in the table on the previous page that many highly processed foods tend to be high GI, meaning that most of the original fibre and nutrients have been stripped away. Conversely, most of the low GI foods on the right are more in their natural state with their nutritional benefits intact.

If there is one thing that nutritionists and the medical profession agree upon, it is that diets rich in fruits, vegetables, whole grains, legumes and low-fat dairy foods are essential for good health and the very large majority of these foods are low GI.

Weight control

High GI foods such as sugary breakfast cereals digest quickly and by mid-morning you are hungry and looking for your next sugar fix.

Conversely, take traditional breakfast porridge oats, the sort many of us haven't had since we were kids. Porridge is low GI and digests more slowly so you are not hungry by the time you get to work. Though you need to avoid adding sugar!

Low GI foods leave you feeling fuller for longer, and enable you to control your appetite and therefore your weight. The next chapter talks about the GI and weight loss in more detail.

Many of Tesco's own-brand products have now been tested to find their GI level and they can be found in the food listing beginning on page 129. They have been divided into three colour-coded categories to indicate whether they are high GI (red), medium GI (yellow) or low GI (green).

Diabetes

Because low GI foods break down more slowly, it means that the supply of glucose into the bloodstream is more gradual and therefore helps moderate blood-sugar levels. Chapter 5 looks at the impact of the GI on health, including diabetes.

WHAT AFFECTS THE GI OF FOODS?

The role of protein and fat

Though the GI is based on carbohydrates, it is also profoundly influenced by protein and fat, both of which act as brakes on your digestive system. Most carbohydrate-based foods also contain both fats and proteins. For instance, some vegetables are a good source of oils, and beans are a good source of protein. When we eat a meal we are usually combining all three food categories in our stomach.

So low GI carbohydrates, low-fat proteins and good fats/oils are the ideal combination of foods for a healthy and nutritious diet.

In the next chapter we will focus on one of the principal health benefits of eating the GI way: weight loss and weight control.

Fibre

Fibre comes in two forms:

- Soluble fibre, which is soluble in water, thickens food, thus slowing down its passage through your digestive tract.
- Insoluble fibre acts as a physical barrier to the digestive enzymes and again slows down the digestive process.

That is one reason why foods high in soluble fibre such as fruits, oats and beans are low GI foods. Foods such as 100% bran breakfast cereals and whole grains are high in insoluble fibre and are low GI.

Impact of cooking and processing

Any processing of food will raise the GI, because processing, usually cooking, is the first step in breaking down food into glucose. This is, in effect, digestion taking place outside your body. For instance, if you have ever had the misfortune to eat a raw potato, you will know that it is almost indigestible and tummy ache is virtually guaranteed. On the other hand, if you eat a baked potato, which is high GI, it digests extremely quickly. In this case the cooking process is the only variable and demonstrates how cooking starts breaking down the starch capsules and fibre, making it easier for your digestive juices to get to work. So when you are cooking foods, especially vegetables, slightly undercook them. This will both help to reduce the loss of vitamins and other essential nutrients as well as keep the GI low.

One other popular food that you should undercook is pasta. Italians call this 'al dente', or 'firm to the bite'. This not only tastes better, but also helps keep the GI lower.

Tinned food products have been subjected to very high temperatures in the canning process to avoid spoilage. Tinned soups are a good example. A tin of soup can sometimes have double the GI when compared to a homemade soup prepared from scratch. While it is sometimes more convenient to use tinned products, especially if you are under time pressure, try to keep these to a minimum and use fresh, dried or frozen products in preference.

Letting your body do the processing is another good reason for always eating the fruit rather than drinking its juice. This way you ensure you're getting all the full benefits, especially fibre, from the fruit rather than buying its highly processed juice. You will also be consuming fewer calories: a glass of orange juice, for instance, contains nearly two and a half times the calories of a fresh orange.

Rice and potatoes

Rice and potatoes are two staples that have unusual GI characteristics. They represent examples of foods that have different GI ratings depending on the type used.

With rice, you should preferably use long-grain or basmati rice rather than the short-grain (glutinous/sticky) variety frequently found in Chinese food. The GI of the latter can be higher by 50% or more.

Potatoes also have a broad GI range. Your best choice is boiled small new potatoes. Large baked potatoes and chips are at the other end of the spectrum. Try not to mash potatoes as this also raises the GI by breaking them down before eating. Remember; let your body do the processing.

SUMMARY

1. Low GI foods are less processed and more nutritious than high GI foods. This benefits your health and reduces your risk of most major diseases including heart disease, stroke, many cancers and diabetes.

2. Low GI foods are more satiating and keep you feeling fuller for longer, which is critical for weight control and weight loss.

3. Low GI foods are helpful in controlling blood-sugar levels, which is essential for managing diseases such as diabetes.

4. Let your body do the processing, not the manufacturer, and don't overcook.

2 Healthy eating for you and your family using the GI Diet

GETTING THE FAMILY INVOLVED

Eating the GI way is not just for you – it's for all the family! Whether you're a busy mum who needs to increase her energy levels, a teenager who wants to shed some puppy fat, a reluctant partner who has developed some unhealthy eating habits over the years or a youngster who is ready to be switched on to a healthy way of eating for life, everyone can reap the benefits from GI.

There are so many advantages to eating the low GI way as a family. First, this is a healthy, nutritious diet. Second, for those members of the family who need to lose weight the advantages are obvious. Third, if you want to avoid cooking three separate meals, then having the whole family eating the same way is clearly the route to go. The GI Diet is not one of those drastic, faddy diets that it's impossible to stay on for more than a few weeks – it's an eating lifestyle that will stand you and your family in good stead for the whole of your lives.

Spouse/partner

Getting your partner or spouse eating the low GI way is important as it's great to have mutual support and encouragement. You both also represent key role models for your children, directly influencing the way they eat.

The best way to get your partner on board is to sit down and discuss your desire to change the way you eat. Point out that, whether or not your partner needs to lose weight, the change to the GI Diet is a healthier way of eating that will provide more energy and reduce the risk of major diseases such as diabetes, heart disease, stroke and cancer. However, as over half the UK population is overweight, there is an odds-on chance that your partner has some pounds to lose.

If you prepare the food but your partner is reluctant to change and give up those favourite high GI foods, then your best option is to introduce more low GI foods to the meals and provide tasty alternatives to high GI choices. This is exactly what you will find in the delicious recipes in the menu plans and recipes on page 84.

You will be amazed how quickly your partner will adapt. Not only because the lower GI choices taste great but also by eating a more nutritional diet, they actually will feel better.

For the serious objector you have two choices:

- Let your partner watch your transformation into a slimmer, more energetic and healthier you, and hear people comment and ask you how you did it. Your partner will soon want to join you and emulate your success!
- Alternatively, you can try the stealth method. Simply adjust the menu and say nothing.

One reader who went on the GI Diet began serving herself and her husband low GI meals for dinner every night without telling him they were based on the GI guidelines. He never even realised he was eating according to the recommendations of a diet plan until he had to have his trousers taken in!

Children

A child's daily nutritional intake affects every aspect of their life. Their behaviour, mood, energy, performances at school and susceptibility to infection and diseases are all affected by what they eat. Many other behaviour issues such as attention deficit disorder could often be helped by diet. There is more detail about this on page 6 of this book.

Do not put children under five years on a low GI diet – they have specific nutritional needs in their early development. For further information on feeding this age group consult your doctor or Tesco pharmacist.

The low GI diet – rich in fruit, vegetables, whole grains, low-fat dairy and meat, nuts and legumes – is ideal for healthy growing children. Just make sure they are getting plenty of good fats in their diet as these are essential for growing bodies. However, you may be wondering how the children are going to co-operate with your new, healthy eating plans. Will they be resistant to change? Or make a stand and demand the foods they're so used to? This could be further complicated by the dynamics of family relationships, which are frequently acted out at mealtimes. Choosing to eat or not gives a child a sense of control. At the same time, mothers rightly consider nutrition and food preparation as one of their key responsibilities towards their family.

The key here is encouragement. Remember, you are introducing a positive new way of looking at food that everyone stands to benefit from in tangible ways, not imposing a draconian diet that will leave everyone famished and unfulfilled! Make it easy for the family to eat healthily. It helps if you set a good example, which is why adopting the GI plan together as a family is the easiest way to get individual family members eating the GI way. Talk things through – focus on the benefits your family will get from changing their eating habits, rather than dwelling on all the things that will no longer be on the menu. Explain how as a result of following the GI plan they will have more energy and, undoubtedly, more confidence.

Also, your children's inherent survival instinct will help determine hunger and appetite. Believe it or not, children are quite capable of regulating their own food intake. They generally have an aversion to new foods, which stems from primitive times when experimenting with new foods could be fatal. However, they will accept them eventually, given sufficient exposure and time. Bear in mind the fact that the more you try to cajole or force food on children, the more likely they are to develop a resistance to eating. Similarly, if they feel deprived, they will have a tendency to overeat. So step back, relax, focus on positive parenting and examine your own food behaviours. Your own behaviour as a role model will have the greatest impact on your child's relationship with food.

The phrase 'Do as I do, not do as I say' could never be more appropriate than when you are trying to get children to eat the right foods. Too often children are excluded from food shopping, meal selection or food preparation. There is no reason why this should be the case. Engage your children in this new venture to get them involved. Explain why and how the family has decided to eat the low GI way. Rather than focusing on weight management, talk about this being a nutritious way of eating aimed at improving the family's health and lifestyle. This is the way the family is going to eat from here on. Make this a big adventure and encourage them to be an active part of it. Remind them that we have a health crisis on our hands mainly because of how we eat. Show them the GI food ratings and you'll be amazed by how quickly they catch on to how it works.

While it is not always practical, the occasional foray with the children to Tesco is a good idea, as they will have an opportunity to learn first-hand why certain food choices are so much better than others. It's an educational opportunity for children. Find out about nutrition while you're stocking up on lots of healthy food together. Explain to your kids what makes certain foods healthier than others and how to combine in a healthy diet. The learning process can be interesting and a lot of fun – and it all starts here.

HOLIDAYS AND CELEBRATIONS

Birthdays, Christmas, Easter and so on all have one thing in common: an abundance of food. It's very easy to over indulge during these times – and it's bound to happen now and again. It's not the end of the world if it does happen, but here are some handy tips to guide you through the holiday period.

Holidays are generally centred around traditional feasts and dishes. But, even so, you don't have to throw the GI guidelines out the window. You can eat the low GI way and still have a fun and festive holiday. If you host the event yourself, you will be able to decide what type of food is served. Think of what you would normally eat during the holiday and look for low GI alternatives.

For example, if you usually have a roast turkey with bread-based stuffing for Christmas, have a roast turkey with wild or basmati rice stuffing instead. If you always make cranberry sauce with sugar, prepare it with a sugar substitute. There is no shortage of low GI vegetables to serve as side dishes, and dessert could be elegant poached pears. You can put on a completely low GI feast without your guests even realising.

If you celebrate the holiday at someone else's home, you will obviously have less control over the menu. You could help out the busy host by offering to bring a vegetable side dish or the dessert – a low GI one of course. Once seated at the holiday table, survey the dishes and try to compose your plate as you would at home: vegetables on half the plate, rice or pasta on one quarter and protein on the other quarter. Pass on the bread rolls and mashed potatoes – have extra vegetables instead. If you wish, you can allow yourself a concession by having a small serving of dessert. If you aren't particularly big on sweets, you might prefer to have a glass of wine instead. Try not to indulge in both.

Cocktail parties can also be fun, low GI occasions. Instead of alcohol, you can have a fruit-juice-based cocktail, a glass of mineral water with a twist of lemon or a diet caffeine-free soft drink. If you really would like an alcoholic beverage, have only one and choose the healthiest option. Red wine is your best bet, or a white wine spritzer made half with wine and half with sparkling water. Be sure to consume any alcohol with food to slow down the rate at which you metabolise it.

Before you go have a low GI meal or snack such as a bowl of low GI cereal with fruit or healthy-eating yoghurt so you won't be tempted to eat too much. Then choose the low GI appetisers and enjoy your time with friends and family.

Just because you are on holiday doesn't mean you shouldn't continue to eat three meals and three snacks daily. In your suitcase, pack some low GI snacks to take which will keep the whole family satisfied, such as nutrition bars, nuts and any other non-perishables. Once there, you can buy low-fat, sugar-free yoghurt, fruit or low-fat cottage cheese to snack on. If you are driving to your destination or are going on a journey, your only option along the motorway may be fast food. If you can, pack some low GI meals and snacks to take with you, so you won't have to stop to eat. Otherwise, we have provided some tips for eating at fast-food outlets on page 72.

FALLING OFF THE WAGON

This is without doubt everyone's major concern and it doesn't need to be. As we stated before, this diet is not a straitjacket. If you can be on the programme for 90% of the time that's just fine. The worst that can happen is that you will delay reaching your weight target by a week or two. This is a real-world way of eating that recognises the realities of social and time pressures, eating on the run and the sheer temptation to binge on occasion. Again, as with food cravings, the GI plan has a built-in warning signal when you go off the rails. After a few weeks eating the low GI way, keeping your blood-sugar levels steady, your body will react with alarm to any sudden onslaught of high GI foods as your blood sugar soars and then plummets, leaving you bloated, tired and irritable. It will be a relief to climb back on board the low GI wagon.

3 Losing or controlling weight with GI

One of the most significant advantages of eating low GI foods is being able to manage your weight. With six out of ten UK adults being overweight, one in five being obese and, even more worrying, a doubling of the number of overweight children in the past twenty years, we have a real epidemic of obesity on our hands; in fact, among western countries, the UK is second only to the US by a whisker. Interestingly, the top four overweight countries are all English-speaking: USA, UK, Australia and Canada!

Here we examine some of the problems with dieting and show how a diet based on the Glycaemic Index can help. For more details on dieting by using the GI, get hold of a copy of *The GI Diet*, *Living the GI Diet* or *The Family GI Diet*, all by Rick Gallop.

PROBLEMS WITH DIETS

Virtually all diets will let you lose weight, so, with over 40% of people on a diet at any one time, why do we have a growing overweight population? The answer is surprisingly simple: people just can't stay on their diets, and there are three basic reasons for this:
• Diets make people feel hungry or deprived.
• Diets can be too complex and time-consuming with counting and measuring of calories (kcals), carbs (carbohydrate portions), points, etc.
• Diets can affect people's health negatively.
That's why it is estimated that 95% of diets ultimately fail.

Eating the low GI way successfully addresses each of these reasons, so if weight loss or weight control is a problem for you or your family – including your children – then read on and find out how and why this will permanently change the way you will eat for the rest of your life. If you have found your previous attempts to lose weight were unsuccessful, you will be delighted with how painless and simple it is for the entire family to lose surplus weight by starting to make intelligent choices about food that will affect their lives from here on in.

Going hungry or feeling deprived

Clearly this is the major stumbling block to anyone trying to stay on a diet. The reason is very simple. All diets work by reducing the number of daily calories (kcals – see page 33) you eat, so you end up eating less than you normally need. For instance, the average woman will need around 1750–2000 calories (kcals) per day to provide the energy her body needs to function. If she takes in only 1500–1750 calories (kcals) in the food she eats, then she will be 250 calories (kcals) short. So, to stop you running out of energy and coming to a grinding halt, your body burns up some of its calorie (kcals) reserves from where they are stored. And we all know that they are stored in those fat cells around our waist and hips! Over time, this usage of calories (kcals) from our fat storage cells leads to a reduction in fat and thus a reduction in weight. This sounds simple enough, but unfortunately your body doesn't like to lose its fat reserves and tells the brain that it is hungry and needs more food.

Where fat fits in

To understand the role of fat, a little background is required. Only a few thousand years ago, a blink of an eye in time from an anthropological viewpoint, we were hunters and gatherers. Agriculture had not been invented and we had to work hard to get our food by hunting it down or gathering it from wild plants. Sometimes game and plants were plentiful and everyone feasted. Sometimes they were scarce, particularly in winter, and everyone fasted. To tide people over the times of famine, our bodies developed an ability to store food as fat: this was increased when things were good and decreased when food was in short supply. So naturally, to avoid possible starvation, our bodies were reluctant to give up the precious fat energy stores without a fight and that is why our hunger pangs are so strong. We may have come a long way in our civilisation since then but our stomachs haven't. Evolution is a lengthy process!

Role of sugar and insulin

The key factor in the process of energy storage and retrieval is insulin. Insulin is a hormone secreted by our pancreas and it does two things extremely well:

- First, it regulates the amount of sugar (glucose) in our bloodstream, removing any excess and storing it as fat.
- Second, it acts as guardian of the fat gates, making our bodies give up their precious fat reserves only reluctantly.

So, controlling insulin is the name of the game. If we stimulate the production of insulin by suddenly dumping a lot of sugar in the bloodstream, it will do its job very efficiently. Soon that sugar 'high', which makes most of us feel great, becomes a sugar 'low' as the insulin rapidly lowers the blood-sugar levels. So then your tummy is looking for its next sugar fix – a low blood-sugar level is the trigger for your appetite. At the same time insulin is resisting giving back its new reserves to curb this appetite.

We need to eat foods that won't over stimulate the production of insulin. And that's how low GI foods can help.

By concentrating on low GI foods that do not raise insulin production, we are able to provide a steady supply of glucose (sugar) to our bloodstream and that means your tummy is not crying out for its next sugar fix.

We have all experienced that mid-afternoon slump when we feel drowsy and lethargic and need a jolt of something to wake us up.

This is a classic example of what happens after you have had a high GI lunch: a bagel or sandwich and maybe a biscuit or muffin to go with your cola. Wham! You get the good short-term feeling of a sugar high (called hyperglycaemia). Insulin kicks in, drains out that excess sugar from your bloodstream to store as fat around your waist and hips, and leaves you with a sugar low (hypoglycaemia). So you grab a Danish to give you an energy boost and your insulin charges in again ... and the yo-yo cycle starts all over again. Sound familiar?

Slow-release low GI foods leave you feeling fuller for longer and not looking for your next sugar fix.

LOSING WEIGHT WITH LOW GI FOODS

A word of warning

As with all good things, there are exceptions. As we discussed earlier, fat also acts as a brake on our digestive system. Fat has twice the calories per gram of carbohydrates or proteins, so a low GI food with a high fat content is clearly not going to help you lose weight.

Similarly, a low GI food may have added sugar. Again, that won't help you lose weight. So, if you are aiming to lose weight and you go to stock up on low GI foods, watch out for products that have a high fat content such as dairy and chocolate. Choose low-fat dairy products, but here is a tip for chocoholics or for kids who can't envisage life without chocolate: look for the high-cocoa versions (such as Tesco *Finest* 72% cocoa). Because of their high chocolate concentration, a couple of squares dissolved slowly will provide as much satisfaction as a whole bar of milk chocolate. Do not make this a regular part of your diet, but use it as a treat!

For products with high sugar content, look for versions where either a sweetener has been added, such as in yoghurt, or where it states 'no sugar added'.

In short, look for low GI foods with low fat (particularly saturated) and low sugar levels. This is not to disparage foods that have a higher GI. Simply, if you want to lose weight, stick to the low or medium GI foods that are low in sugar and saturated fat. See GI food listings, pages 129–38.

Meals and snacks

Lastly and most importantly comes the matter of when, and how often, you should be eating your low GI meals. As we discussed earlier, it is important to keep your tummy busy so that it's not looking for its next meal. We recommend three main meals: breakfast, lunch and dinner. Also three snacks: mid-morning, mid-afternoon and before bedtime.

BREAKFAST

This is the most important meal because most of us won't have eaten since dinner the night before. If you miss breakfast, then you could be without food for up to sixteen hours – particularly bad news for children with a busy school day ahead of them. The result is that you load up on snacks and pig out at other meals. So make sure you have a good low GI breakfast containing low GI carbs, little saturated fat and low-fat protein. Porridge is the ultimate breakfast for each and every family member, and one of the best choices you can make while following the GI Diet. Other breakfast suggestions and recipes can be found on pages 84–6.

LUNCH

Most of us eat lunch outside the home, so eating the low GI way can be a problem. Packed lunches are a wonderful option which will serve you (at work) and your children (at school or at play) equally well. We have some suggestions in Chapter 7 on eating outside the home (see page 70 as to how you can make your packed lunch a low GI one). Should you prefer, or should you have to eat out, there are suggestions on how to eat the low GI way at restaurants, fast-food and takeaway outlets.

DINNER

Dinner is traditionally the main meal of the day and in general we tend to have more time for preparing and enjoying the meal. It's important to make time for a proper family dinner at least two or three times a week. This way, you will know that your family are eating healthily, and it will encourage and establish healthy eating habits.

A typical dinner consists of three parts: meat or seafood; potato, pasta or rice; and vegetables. Together these foods provide proteins, fats and carbohydrates along with other minerals and vitamins essential to our health. Some people add a starter or, more commonly, a dessert.

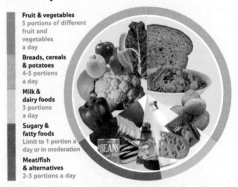

Fruit & vegetables
5 portions of different fruit and vegetables a day

Breads, cereals & potatoes
4-5 portions a day

Milk & dairy foods
3 portions a day

Sugary & fatty foods
Limit to 1 portion a day or in moderation

Meat/fish & alternatives
2-3 portions a day

The Government's Balance of Good Health (National Food Guide) recommends that anyone over the age of five should divide the balance of these different food groups into five parts (see the diagram on page 29). If you are aiming to lose weight, you should visualise your plate with one half containing at least two vegetables; one quarter potato, rice or pasta; and the other quarter, meat or seafood (for vegetarians, eggs, Quorn, tofu and beans). Whenever possible it is good to add a side salad.

For choices of meats, seafood, vegetables, pasta and rice, see Chapter 4 on Shopping, page 42.

Although desserts can be a problem when eating out, they should form an integral part of your meal when at home, as they can provide other sources of vitamins and minerals. Kids, in particular, tend to adore desserts, and luckily there is a broad range of lower GI dessert options that taste great, as well as being good for them. Most fruits and low-fat dairy foods are ideal choices.

SNACKS

Three low GI snacks a day require a little planning and we list some suggestions below. Try and eat balanced snacks, i.e. those containing some carbs, fat and protein. This is particularly important if you are concerned about your blood-sugar levels, especially if you have, or are at risk of having, type II diabetes (see page 55).

SNACK SUGGESTIONS*

Nuts – almonds, hazelnuts

Fresh fruit – apple, orange, grapefruit

Vegetables – celery, carrots, sliced bell peppers

Low-fat dairy foods – cottage cheese, cheese (Healthy Living Low Fat Cheese Spread), yoghurt

Nutrition (cereal) bars

High-bran cereals – All Bran

Porridge

* Other snack recipes can be found in *Living the GI Diet*

BEVERAGES

- **Water:** As water makes up 50–70% of our body, it is not surprising that your liquid intake is so important. Water facilitates the digestive process, helps flush out waste and toxins and is part of a healthy diet. Most nutritionists recommend eight glasses of water a day. A good rule of thumb is to have a 250ml glass of water before each meal or snack. Having your stomach partly filled with liquid makes you feel full more quickly, thus reducing the temptation to overeat. Get your children used to drinking plenty of water now and they will carry this fantastic habit with them into later life.

- **Skimmed milk:** This is an ideal low GI food. Try to drink at least one glass a day, preferably two. If you want a quick boost to your protein input, this is an easy solution which provides a good source of calcium.

- **Coffee:** The problem with coffee is caffeine and the cravings it can create. Caffeine stimulates the production of insulin. As we know, insulin reduces blood-sugar levels, which increases your appetite. This is not helpful when we are trying our best to keep our appetite under control. So avoid coffee if you are dieting. Don't despair; there are some delicious decaffeinated coffees available. If a jolt of Java is essential to your survival, then go for it, but make it one cup a day maximum.

- **Tea:** Tea has much less caffeine than coffee and has the added bonus of flavonoids (antioxidants), which are beneficial to heart health. Green tea is even better. So, tea in moderation is just fine.

- **Fruit drinks/juices:** These are high in sugar and are high GI. Avoid these if you wish to lose weight. Fruit juices and squash have a lower GI but are still calorie dense. Always eat the fruit (or vegetable) rather than drink its juice. You'll get more fibre nutrient value, a lower GI and fewer calories. Encourage your children to choose no-added-sugar versions of juice or squash and dilute with plenty of water, which makes the drinks more thirst-quenching, too.

- **Alcohol:** Alcohol should definitely be avoided if you wish to lose weight. Because alcohol metabolises so quickly it creates a short-term high, but it actually lowers your blood sugar. And, unfortunately, the buzz from alcohol means you don't always want to stop after one drink. If you are drinking alcohol remember that the safe upper limits for men and women are four and three units per day respectively. Don't multiply this by seven and assume it to be a safe weekly intake. Aim to have one or two alcohol-free days each week. For reference, a 'unit' is equivalent to:
  - 1 small glass (125ml) of 9% ABV wine (pub measures are generally larger than this – 175ml and even 250ml) and most wines nowadays are higher in alcohol, so these will contain more units per glass)
  - half a pint of ordinary strength (3%) lager or bitter
  - single measure of spirits or aperitifs (home measures tend to be larger!).

Reading labels

To help you make better food choices, Tesco are putting new labels on the front of their packs to show the amount of calories, sugar, fat, saturates and salt you'll consume by eating a serving of the food. The label also shows how much of your Guideline Daily Amount (GDA) the food provides. The percentage GDA will help you make a judgement on where a product fits in with your diet.

Calories	Sugar	Fat	Saturates	Salt
114	6.9g	3.8g	0.4g	1.8g
6%	8%	6%	2%	30%

The nutritional panel on the following page can be found on the back of packs.

Pak choi, baby corn, spring onion, sweet pepper and mangetout.

Ingredients

Pak Choi (36%), Baby Corn (16%), Sweet Pepper (16%), Spring Onion (16%), Mangetout (16%).

Nutrition

Typical Composition	A 95g (3½oz) serving provides	100g (3½oz) provide
Energy	127kJ	133kJ
	30kcal	32kcal
Protein	2.0g	2.1g
Carbohydrate	3.8g	4.0g
of which sugars	3.4g	3.6g
Fat	0.8g	0.8g
of which saturates	trace	trace
Fibre	2.2g	2.3g
Sodium	trace	trace

This pack contains 2 servings.
A serving (95g) contains the equivalent of trace of salt.

Guideline daily amounts for an average adult

	Guideline daily amount	Each 95g serving	% guideline daily amount
Calories	2000kcal	30kcal	2%
Sugar	90g	3.4g	4%
Fat	70g	0.8g	1%
Saturated fat	20g	trace	<1%
Salt	6g	trace	<1%

For further information, visit:
www.tesco.com/health

Free from
• Nuts.

Stir fry – high heat   4 mins
• Remove all packaging.
• All appliances vary, these are guidelines only.
• Not suitable for microwave cooking.
• Heat 1 x 15ml (1tbsp) of oil in a wok or frying pan.
• Add contents of pack.
• Stir fry over a medium/high heat for 4 minutes, stirring continuously.
• Serve immediately.

Storage
• Keep refrigerated.
• Use by: see front of pack.
• Not suitable for home freezing.

Our promise
We are happy to refund or replace any Tesco product which falls below the high standard you expect. Just ask any member of staff. This does not affect your statutory rights.

We are here to help:
Tesco Stores Ltd., Cheshunt EN8 9SL U.K.
Freephone 0800 50 55 55
www.tesco.com

190g

Packed for Tesco Stores Ltd., Cheshunt, EN8 9SL U.K. ©Tesco 2005. SCHM

Let's examine the information on a typical food label. The first things to look for are:

• **Serving size**: Check the stated serving size.

When you are comparing brands of any type of food, make sure you are comparing the same serving sizes. For example, look at each per 100g.

• **Calories (kcals)**: Obviously, if you are intending to lose weight, then this is a key criterion in your selection of brands. Calories are usually referred to as kcals on labels. Again, when you are comparing brands, this is the first item to check, as it often flags up possible problems with fat and sugar levels.

• **Fat**: Here we are looking for low-fat brands, e.g. Tesco Healthy Living, but, more importantly, those with the lowest saturated fat levels.

• **Fibre**: this is really critical in the low GI programme as the GI of foods is significantly affected by its fibrous content. Fibrous foods have a lower GI, so when you are comparing brands, look for those with higher fibre levels.

• **Salt**: Salt has a major impact on blood pressure. If you have any major risk factors for heart disease and stroke, such as being overweight, having high blood pressure (hypertension), or a genetic predisposition to these diseases, you should pay close attention to the sodium or salt content.

• **Sugar**: Again, if losing weight is your main concern, sugar levels are important to watch.

33

BEST BUY

Look on the label for:

- low or medium GI rating (see GI food lists on pages 129–38)
- low sugar levels
- lower fat content, particularly saturated fats
- higher fibre levels
- and, if you are at risk of heart disease or stroke, then look for low salt (sodium).

RECOMMENDED SERVING SIZES FOR DIETING

FOODS	PORTION RECOMMENDED
Low GI breads (which have at least 2½–3g fibre per slice)	1 slice (28g/1oz)
Low GI cereals	60g (2oz)
Nuts (unsalted)	8–10
Margarine (reduced fat)	2 tsp
Meat, seafood, poultry (the size of a pack of cards)	120g (4oz)
Olive/rapeseed oil	1 tsp
Olives	4–5
Pasta	40g (1⅓oz) uncooked
Potatoes (boiled, new)	2–3
Rice (long grain, basmati)	50g (1¼oz) uncooked

Portions and serving sizes

Another big advantage of eating the low GI way is that, on the whole, there are no recommended serving sizes. This is not a deprivation diet. For the most part you can eat as much of the low GI foods as you like. There are a few exceptions – those that have a higher fat or calorie content, for example, which are listed below.

What is required is a large dose of common sense so you don't start eating twelve apples a day or a litre of low-fat yoghurt at one sitting. We don't recommend that you go overboard on quantities of anything. Moderation is the keyword.

Two-step plan

In Rick Gallop's *The GI Diet*, he has developed two steps or phases in his weight-control programme:

STEP 1

This is the weight-loss period when you will lose those pounds painlessly without going hungry and feeling deprived. Here you will focus on low GI foods that are also low in fat and sugar. This doesn't mean you can't have the occasional fling. Falling off the wagon, while not encouraged, is acceptable, as this diet is not a straitjacket. Try to eat the low GI way 90% of the time and you will be doing fine. The occasional lapse at worst will only delay you achieving your target weight level by a week or two.

STEP 2

This is the maintenance phase and how you will eat for the rest of your life! Here you are encouraged to add more medium GI foods to your diet and you may increase the above serving sizes by up to 50%. This is also a time to reward yourself for achieving your target weight by adding some of the forbidden foods such as 70% cocoa chocolate or a glass of wine (preferably red) with your dinner. Wine has been demonstrated to be beneficial to heart health but do not make the assumption that, if one glass is good for you, two will be even better and so on! One glass per day is your best option.

A word of warning. By this time your new leaner body will require fewer calories to function as you have less weight to carry around, and it has also learned how to use calories more efficiently while you've been reducing your calorie input. So you don't need to make any significant changes to your diet to maintain your new weight. Just stick to low and medium GI foods that are low in fat, particularly saturated fat, and sugar.

One of the amazing benefits you will feel with your new body is your increased energy level. Not really surprising if you realise how much extra weight you used to carry around. A good way to understand this is to pack a knapsack full of books (your old diet books!) weighing about the same as the weight you have lost. Carry it around the house for an hour one evening and then put it down. That is what you have been carrying around all the time! No wonder you had no energy, sore joints and found it painful to exercise. Keep that knapsack handy and pick it up from time to time to use as a motivator and reminder.

HOW MUCH WEIGHT SHOULD I LOSE?

Body Mass Index
Everyone has their own particular body make-up, metabolism and genes so there are no absolute rules for how much you should weigh. The nearest to an international standard is the Body Mass Index (BMI) which measures your weight against your height. You can calculate your BMI by dividing your weight in kilograms by your height in metres squared. For example, if you weigh 60kg and you are 1.60m tall, then 60 ÷ (1.60 x 1.60) = 23.4. To find your BMI quickly, use the chart on p38–9. Find your height on the horizontal row at the top and your weight on the vertical column on the left. Your BMI is where the two intersect.

If your BMI falls between 19 and 24, your weight is within the acceptable norm; 25–29 is viewed as overweight; and 30+ as obese. With a bit of extra calculation, you can work out what would be an acceptable weight for your height and that should then indicate how much weight you need to lose.

Women have a lower muscle mass and smaller frame than men, so women might want to target towards the lower end of the range while men should generally target the higher end. However, if you are pregnant, breastfeeding, under eighteen, elderly, chronically ill or of a muscular build, then these ratings do not apply to you. For those over 65, we suggest you allow an extra 4.5kg (10lb) to help protect you in case of a fall or as an extra energy reserve should you suffer a long debilitating illness.

As we've said before, use this only as a guide, not as an absolute number. Nevertheless, it's a good general measure and the only one that has been accepted as an international standard.

Waist measurement

The other measurement you should concern yourself with is your waist measurement. This is an even better predictor of your health than is your weight. Abdominal fat is more than just an added weight problem. Recent research has shown that abdominal fat acts almost like a separate organ in the body, but this 'organ' is destructive – it releases harmful proteins and free fatty acids into the rest of the body and this can increase your risk of heart disease, stroke, cancer and diabetes. Doctors describe people with abdominal fat as apple-shaped.

If you are female and have a waist measurement of 88cm+ (32in+), or male with a waist measurement of 93cm (37in+), you are at risk of endangering your health. If this measurement is 93cm+ (35in+) for women and 100cm+ (40in+) for men, then you are at serious risk of heart disease, stroke, many cancers and diabetes.

STONES	LBS	POUNDS	KILOS	4'6" / 137	4'8" / 142	4'10" / 147	5'0" / 152	5'2" / 157	5'3" / 160	5'4" / 163	5'5" / 165	5'6" / 168	5'7" / 170	5'8" / 173	5'9" / 175	5'10" / 178	5'11" / 180	6'0" / 183	6'2" / 188	6'4" / 193	6'6" / 198	6'8" / 203
6	7	91	41	22.0	20.4	19.0	17.8	16.6	16.1	15.6	15.1	14.7	14.3	13.8	13.4	13.1	12.7	12.3	11.7	11.1	10.5	10.0
6	10	94	43	22.7	21.1	19.6	18.4	17.2	16.7	16.1	15.6	15.2	14.7	14.3	13.9	13.5	13.1	12.7	12.1	11.4	10.9	10.3
7	0	98	44	23.7	22.0	20.5	19.1	17.9	17.4	16.8	16.3	15.8	15.3	14.9	14.5	14.1	13.7	13.3	12.6	11.9	11.3	10.8
7	3	101	46	24.4	22.6	21.1	19.7	18.5	17.9	17.3	16.8	16.3	15.8	15.4	14.9	14.5	14.1	13.7	13.0	12.3	11.7	11.1
7	7	105	48	25.4	23.5	21.9	20.5	19.2	18.6	18.0	17.5	16.9	16.4	16.0	15.5	15.1	14.6	14.2	13.5	12.8	12.1	11.5
7	10	108	49	26.1	24.2	22.6	21.1	19.8	19.1	18.5	18.0	17.4	16.9	16.4	15.9	15.5	15.1	14.6	13.9	13.1	12.5	11.9
8	0	112	51	27.1	25.1	23.4	21.9	20.5	19.8	19.2	18.6	18.1	17.5	17.0	16.5	16.1	15.6	15.2	14.4	13.6	12.9	12.3
8	3	115	52	27.8	25.8	24.0	22.5	21.0	20.4	19.7	19.1	18.6	18.0	17.5	17.0	16.5	16.0	15.6	14.8	14.0	13.3	12.6
8	7	119	54	28.8	26.7	24.9	23.2	21.8	21.1	20.4	19.8	19.2	18.6	18.1	17.6	17.1	16.6	16.1	15.3	14.5	13.8	13.1
8	10	122	55	29.5	27.4	25.5	23.8	22.3	21.6	20.9	20.3	19.7	19.1	18.5	18.0	17.5	17.0	16.5	15.7	14.9	14.1	13.4
9	0	129	59	31.2	28.9	27.0	25.2	23.6	22.9	22.1	21.5	20.8	20.2	19.6	19.0	18.5	18.0	17.5	16.6	15.7	14.9	14.2
9	7	133	60	32.1	29.8	27.8	26.0	24.3	23.6	22.8	22.1	21.5	20.8	20.2	19.6	19.1	18.5	18.0	17.1	16.2	15.4	14.6
9	10	136	62	32.9	30.5	28.4	26.6	24.9	24.1	23.3	22.6	22.0	21.3	20.7	20.1	19.5	19.0	18.4	17.5	16.6	15.7	14.9
10	0	140	64	33.8	31.4	29.3	27.3	25.6	24.8	24.0	23.3	22.6	21.9	21.3	20.7	20.1	19.5	19.0	18.0	17.0	16.2	15.4
10	3	143	65	34.6	32.1	29.9	27.9	26.2	25.3	24.5	23.8	23.1	22.4	21.7	21.1	20.5	19.9	19.4	18.4	17.4	16.5	15.7
10	7	147	67	35.5	33.0	30.7	28.7	26.9	26.0	25.2	24.5	23.7	23.0	22.4	21.7	21.1	20.5	19.9	18.9	17.9	17.0	16.1
10	10	150	68	36.3	33.6	31.3	29.3	27.4	26.5	25.7	25.0	24.2	23.5	22.8	22.1	21.5	20.9	20.3	19.3	18.3	17.3	16.5
11	0	154	70	37.2	34.5	32.2	30.1	28.2	27.3	26.4	25.6	24.9	24.1	23.4	22.7	22.1	21.5	20.9	19.8	18.7	17.8	16.9
11	3	157	71	37.9	35.2	32.8	30.7	28.7	27.8	26.9	26.1	25.3	24.6	23.9	23.2	22.5	21.9	21.3	20.2	19.1	18.1	17.2
11	7	161	73	38.9	36.1	33.6	31.4	29.4	28.5	27.6	26.8	26.0	25.2	24.5	23.8	23.1	22.5	21.8	20.7	19.6	18.6	17.7
11	10	164	74	39.6	36.7	34.3	32.0	30.0	29.1	28.2	27.3	26.5	25.7	24.9	24.2	23.5	22.9	22.2	21.1	20.0	19.0	18.0
12	0	168	76	40.6	37.7	35.1	32.8	30.7	29.8	28.8	28.0	27.1	26.3	25.5	24.8	24.1	23.4	22.8	21.6	20.4	19.4	18.5
12	3	171	78	41.3	38.3	35.7	33.4	31.3	30.3	29.4	28.5	27.6	26.8	26.0	25.3	24.5	23.8	23.2	22.0	20.8	19.8	18.8
12	7	175	79	42.3	39.2	36.6	34.2	32.0	31.0	30.0	29.1	28.2	27.4	26.6	25.8	25.1	24.4	23.7	22.5	21.3	20.2	19.2

st	lb	lbs	kg																				
12	10	178	81	19.6	20.6	21.7	22.9	24.1	25.5	26.3	27.1	27.9	28.7	29.6	30.6	31.5	32.6	34.8	37.2	39.9	43.0						
13	0	182	83	20.0	21.0	22.2	23.4	24.7	26.1	26.9	27.7	28.5	29.4	30.3	31.2	32.2	33.3	35.5	38.0	40.8	44.0						
13	3	185	84	20.3	21.4	22.5	23.8	25.1	26.5	27.3	28.1	29.0	29.9	30.8	31.8	32.8	33.8	36.1	38.7	41.5	44.7						
13	7	189	86	20.8	21.8	23.0	24.3	25.6	27.1	27.9	28.7	29.6	30.5	31.5	32.4	33.5	34.6	36.9	39.5	42.4	45.7						
13	10	192	87	21.1	22.2	23.4	24.7	26.0	27.5	28.4	29.2	30.1	31.0	31.9	33.0	34.0	35.1	37.5	40.1	43.0	46.4						
14	0	196	89	21.5	22.6	23.9	25.2	26.6	28.1	28.9	29.8	30.7	31.6	32.6	33.6	34.7	35.8	38.3	41.0	43.9	47.4						
14	3	199	90	21.9	23.0	24.2	25.5	27.0	28.6	29.4	30.3	31.2	32.1	33.1	34.2	35.3	36.4	38.9	41.6	44.6	48.1						
14	7	203	92	22.3	23.5	24.7	26.1	27.5	29.1	30.0	30.9	31.8	32.8	33.8	34.8	36.0	37.1	39.6	42.4	45.5	49.1						
14	10	206	93	22.6	23.8	25.1	26.4	27.9	29.6	30.4	31.3	32.3	33.2	34.3	35.4	36.5	37.7	40.2	43.1	46.2	49.8						
15	0	210	95	23.1	24.3	25.6	27.0	28.5	30.1	31.0	31.9	32.9	33.9	34.9	36.0	37.2	38.4	41.0	43.9	47.1	50.8						
15	3	213	97	23.4	24.6	25.9	27.3	28.9	30.6	31.5	32.4	33.4	34.4	35.4	36.6	37.7	39.0	41.6	44.5	47.8	51.5						
15	7	217	98	23.8	25.1	26.4	27.9	29.4	31.1	32.0	33.0	34.0	35.0	36.1	37.2	38.4	39.7	42.4	45.4	48.6	52.4						
15	10	220	100	24.2	25.4	26.8	28.2	29.8	31.6	32.5	33.5	34.5	35.5	36.6	37.8	39.0	40.2	43.0	46.0	49.3	53.2						
16	0	224	102	24.6	25.9	27.3	28.8	30.4	32.1	33.1	34.1	35.1	36.2	37.3	38.4	39.7	41.0	43.7	46.8	50.2	54.1						
16	3	227	103	24.9	26.2	27.6	29.1	30.8	32.6	33.5	34.5	35.6	36.6	37.8	39.0	40.2	41.5	44.3	47.4	50.9	54.9						
16	7	231	105	25.4	26.7	28.1	29.7	31.3	33.1	34.1	35.1	36.2	37.3	38.4	39.7	40.9	42.2	45.1	48.3	51.8	55.8						
16	10	234	106	25.7	27.0	28.5	30.0	31.7	33.6	34.6	35.6	36.6	37.8	38.9	40.2	41.5	42.8	45.7	48.9	52.5	56.6						
17	0	238	108	26.1	27.5	29.0	30.6	32.3	34.1	35.1	36.2	37.3	38.4	39.6	40.9	42.2	43.5	46.5	49.7	53.4	57.5						
17	7	245	111	26.9	28.3	29.8	31.4	33.2	35.1	36.1	37.3	38.3	39.5	40.7	42.0	43.3	44.8	47.8	51.2	54.9	59.0						
18	0	252	114	27.6	29.1	30.5	32.3	34.1	36.1	37.2	38.3	39.4	40.6	41.9	43.2	44.6	46.0	49.2	52.6	56.4	60.7						
18	7	259	117	28.4	29.9	31.5	33.2	35.1	37.1	38.2	39.3	40.5	41.8	43.0	44.4	45.8	47.3	50.5	54.1	58.0	62.4						
19	0	266	120	29.2	30.7	32.3	34.1	36.0	38.1	39.2	40.4	41.6	42.9	44.2	45.6	47.1	48.6	51.9	55.5	59.6	64.1						
19	7	273	123	29.9	31.5	33.2	35.0	37.0	39.1	40.3	41.5	42.7	44.0	45.4	46.8	48.3	49.9	53.3	57.0	61.2	65.8						
20	0	280	126	30.7	32.3	34.0	35.9	37.9	40.1	41.3	42.5	43.8	45.1	46.5	48.0	49.5	51.2	54.6	58.5	62.7	67.5						

To measure your waist put a tape measure around your waist at navel level till it fits snugly and is not cutting into your flesh. Do not adopt the walk-down-the-beach-suck-in-your-tummy routine! Just stand naturally. There's no point in trying to fudge the numbers because the only person you're kidding is yourself.

HOW LONG SHOULD IT TAKE?

This is inevitably the question that follows, 'How much should I lose?'

If you are planning to lose up to 10% of your body weight (e.g. you weigh 63.6kg (10 stones) and want to lose 6.3kg (1 stone)) then you should plan on losing an average of 450g (1lb) per week. We say average, because you never lose weight in a straight line. The pattern is to lose weight more quickly at the start of the diet, followed by a series of drops and plateaux. The closer you get to your target weight, the slower your weight loss. So for a 6.3kg (1 stone) loss, assume about fourteen weeks.

If you have more than 10% to lose, the good news is that you will lose more than 450g (1lb) on average a week. This is simply because your larger body requires more calories just to keep operating than someone who is lighter. For example, Mary weighs 95.4kg (15 stones) with a BMI of 34 and requires about 2700 calories a day just to keep her body operating. Jane, who is the same height but weighs 70kg (11 stones) with a BMI of 26, only needs 2000 calories per day. A typical calorie level for a low GI diet is 1500 calories per day. So Mary will be reducing her calorie intake by 1200 calories per day, which equals a weight loss of over 1kg (21/2lb) per week. Jane on the other hand has a shortfall of only 500 calories per day, which equals a weight loss of 450g (1lb) per week.

These are only approximate figures but will give you some idea of what you should expect.

SUMMARY

1. Be super positive about the healthy eating changes you are introducing into the household.

2. Invite your partner and children to get involved in every step of the process.

3. For those who wish to lose weight, record current weights and waist measurements. Set target weights. Try the knapsack test.

4. Clear the larder and fridge of all high GI foods and replace with low GI foods. (See Chapter 4 on shopping.)

5. Only eat low GI products that are low in fat, especially saturated fat, and low in sugar. Read the label!

6. Make exercise an integral part of the family's life. See Chapter 6 for inspiration.

7. Pack your own lower-GI snacks when travelling.

4 Shopping

Now that you are convinced that eating the low GI way is the way to go, you're ready to hit your nearest Tesco – hopefully with one or more family members in tow. Involving your children in the shopping process can be a highly positive experience. Encourage them to open their eyes and take in all the information around them that they probably never noticed before. For example, urge them to take a look at the food ingredients on labels. Once they realise what actually goes into a lot of products, they will soon start erring on the side of healthy eating as a matter of course! Point out all the weird and wonderful fruit and vegetables that exist from around the world. The world is our oyster when it comes to food.

But before you set out with your book and shopping list in hand, there are a couple of preliminary steps:

• **Clear out the larder**. Almost certainly your cupboards and fridge will contain a selection of high GI foods. So to make a clean break with your unhealthy past and to avoid future temptations, clear them out! If the thought of throwing them in the dustbin makes you feel guilty, then donate them to your local charity or skinny neighbours. It will be a clear sign to the family that changes are on the way and everyone will soon be eating in a new, healthy and nutritious way.

• **Eat before you shop**. One of the worst mistakes you can make is to go shopping on an empty stomach. The result will be that you will be more tempted to buy those high GI, fat- and sugar-rich foods, however good your original intentions. The first few times you shop the low GI way will require a little more time and concentration. It is not a time to be distracted by an empty tummy. Soon it will become second nature and your new eating patterns will be well established – you will be less likely to be distracted by hunger pangs. If you're eating the low GI way, then in any case hunger pangs will be a thing of the past!

You have now arrived at Tesco with your shopping list and book in hand with a full stomach. We propose to take you section by section through the store giving you some guidelines for making the right GI choices.

All of the low GI foods listed in this chapter are also low in saturated fat and calories. If you want to lose or control your weight, then these are your best choices.

VEGETABLES

Vegetables are a low GI wonderland. Virtually all vegetables are low GI and high in fibre, nutrients, minerals and vitamins. The only general exceptions are root vegetables (check listings on page 130). They also count towards your '5-a-day' target. As we discussed earlier, cooking raises the GI of foods and also reduces some of the nutrient content. So try eating them raw with a tasty low-fat dip as a snack; if you do need to cook them, use as little water as possible and undercook – microwaving is excellent for preparing vegetables. Remember, cooking is the first step in the digestive process of breaking down food. The more processing that goes on outside your body, the less your digestive system is left to do. And, as we discussed earlier, the more processing your body has to do, the better. Keeping your digestive system busy means it is not looking for its next meal!

Just look at the incredible range of vegetables that are available at Tesco from all over the world. Unfortunately most of us limit our choices to a narrow selection. So break with tradition, live a little and choose some that you've never tried before.

The only vegetables that have a medium or high GI are certain root vegetables such as potatoes, turnips and beetroot. If you are trying to lose weight, avoid these in Step 1. The main exceptions are carrots and new potatoes. As we discussed on page 16, it is the type of potato you eat and how you prepare it that counts. Boiled small new potatoes are your best bet.

FRUITS

Fresh

Virtually all fresh fruits are low GI and also count towards your '5-a-day' target. A few exceptions are those with particularly high sugar and low fibre levels, which digest quickly resulting in a high GI rating. Melons are a good example of this.

Fruits are an excellent source of fibre, vitamins and minerals, all of which are essential for good health. They should form a cornerstone of your diet.

Frozen, bottled, canned, dried

As fresh fruits and vegetables can be expensive out of season, then your next best option is frozen. Frozen fruit and vegetables have virtually the same nutritional value as fresh fruit and vegetables and, when bought in bulk, can be reasonably inexpensive.

Bottled and canned foods are a less advantageous choice as the bottling/canning process requires high temperatures to avoid spoilage. This not only destroys some of the nutritional value but also raises the GI of the fruit. If you do buy canned fruit or vegetables, always drain off the water or juice first as they sometimes contain added sugar. Choose those that are tinned in natural juice rather than syrup.

Many dried fruits are red light as they are very high in sugar. However, dried apricots, cranberries, apples and prunes are yellow light. All dried fruits are acceptable to use in modest quantities as baking ingredients to enhance flavour. The Tesco Wholefoods range offers some natural healthy choices.

Juices

The golden rule is to eat the fruit rather than drink the juice. The whole fruit has a lower GI, fewer calories and more fibre and nutrition than the processed juice. Though the traditional breakfast orange juice can be a hard habit to break, it's worth doing.

MEAT, SOYA, POULTRY, SEAFOOD, MYCOPROTEIN

Meat/soya

Most meats contain fat, especially saturated fat, so it's important to select meats that have had all the visible fat trimmed and that are also intrinsically lean, e.g. Healthy Living Chicken, Pork or Beef. Simply trimming visible fat can reduce the amount of fat by an average of 50%. Round or loin cuts are the best for a lean choice. Processed meats such as salami can be high in fat and salt, and are not your best choices.

Soya-based foods such as tofu, mycoprotein (e.g. Quorn) and TVP (textured vegetable protein) are high in protein, low in saturated fat and are good for a healthy heart. An excellent choice whether you are vegetarian or not.

Remember, the serving size is 115g (4oz) or about the size of a pack of cards or the palm of your hand.

Poultry – chicken and turkey (without skin)

The traditional benchmark for low-fat protein is skinless chicken or turkey breast. Skin removal is critical with all poultry. Dark meat (thigh, leg), duck and goose are higher in saturated fat.

In Step 1 (weight-loss phase) skinless chicken and turkey should be your preferred source of protein. They are relatively inexpensive and can be prepared in a variety of interesting ways from stir-fries to chicken salads.

Seafood

All fish and shellfish are excellent choices. Here is an opportunity to explore the wonderful world of seafood outside the traditional family favourites: salmon and tuna. There is a wide variety available at Tesco from the fish counter or in pre-packaged form. One caution, seafood that is breaded or battered is not your best choice.

From a health standpoint, oily fish, such as salmon, mackerel or trout, is rich in omega-3, an oil that is beneficial against heart disease and stroke.

CEREAL GRAINS

Whole grains with all the nutrition and fibre intact are, in general, low GI, but remember that rice is one of the grains where the GI can range from high to low. Basmati and long grain rice are good choices. Brown and wild rice, although usually more expensive, are an even better choice, as they are less processed and contain more nutrients and fibre. However, short grain rice that is glutinous and sticks together (similar to that served in Chinese restaurants or the Italian risotto rice) is not recommended.

SUGARS/SWEETENERS/FRUIT SPREADS

Sugars
Sugar and derivatives such as golden syrup and brown sugar are all high GI.

Sweeteners
The better choice is to go for one of the latest sweeteners, some of which are based on sugar (sucralose) and measure exactly like sugar. There are several excellent, safe sugar substitutes on the market and they have been approved by all Western government health agencies. If you are sensitive to aspartame, there are other great choices.

Fruit spreads
These can be used as straightforward spreads on bread/toast or can be used as flavour enhancers with cereals, porridge and low-fat dairy products such as yoghurt, sour cream and cottage cheese.

Your best choices are spreads that contain extra fruit and low amounts of added sugar – or preferably none. The clue is in the product contents listings on the label. If sugar is the first ingredient then this is not your best choice if you're trying to lose weight.

BEANS (LEGUMES)

Beans (or legumes) are almost the perfect food. Rich in protein, fibre and low in fat, they are a star in the low GI food listings. Soya beans in particular are valuable to vegetarians as a source of protein and are very heart healthy.

Fresh, frozen or dried beans are your best choice. Canned beans can have a GI up to 50% higher because of the high temperatures used in the canning process to avoid spoilage. However, they still fall into the low to moderate GI range, albeit at the higher end. Watch out for beans with added meat, sugar or molasses. These are not your best choices. Make beans a priority in your low GI shopping list.

CONDIMENTS/SEASONINGS

Many condiments are low GI, such as mustard and horseradish. Read the list of ingredients and watch out for sugar or other natural sweeteners such as honey and brown sugar. Ketchup and brown sauce have high sugar content, so use them sparingly.

FATS/OILS/DRESSINGS

Fat is an essential part of a healthy diet. The issue is eating the right type of fat. (See pages 8–10.)

The good fats and oils are vegetable-based and the gold star award goes to rapeseed oil and olive oil. These should be your preferred choices.

Dressings should be low fat. You can make your own simple low GI dressing by squeezing the juice of a lemon onto your meal.

As acid reduces the GI level of a meal, in that it slows the digestive process, low fat or reduced fat vinaigrette dressing makes an ideal choice.

NUTS AND SEEDS

Nuts and seeds, such as those in the Tesco Wholefoods range, are an excellent source of good fats and protein. Some nuts have more monounsaturated (best) fat than others. Remember that all nuts are calorie dense so limit your quantities (typically 8–10 nuts per serving). It is very easy to sit in front of the TV and consume quite unconsciously a bowl of nuts which, incidentally, equals your total calorie needs for an entire day!

While 100% nut butters, such as peanut butter, have a low GI and contain good fats, they are very high in calories so should be used in very limited quantities. If you can restrain yourself to 1 tablespoon, you can have this as an occasional treat in Step 1. Only 100% peanut brands qualify, as other versions contain fillers such as sugar, starches or hydrogenated oils.

PASTA

Most durum wheat pastas are low to medium GI, especially the wholemeal variety. Just watch the quantity (a maximum of 115g /4oz – or 40g/1⅓oz, if dieting – uncooked) and always slightly undercook – al dente. All pastas with cheese or meat fillings or which are pre-packaged or tinned are not good choices if you are trying to lose weight.

Pasta sauces
Tomato paste sauces that are low in sugar are the best choice. Tomato sauce is also rich in lycopene, which has been shown to reduce the risk of prostate cancer.

SNACKS

For those trying to lose weight we recommend three snacks a day, so this is an important section, but loaded with aisles of temptation!

Fortunately there are many excellent choices ranging from low-fat dairy products to nutrition (cereal) bars (see next page), fruit and nuts. Snacks are also important for growing children who expend masses of energy during the day.

SOUPS

Soups are useful for reducing the amount of food you eat during the rest of the meal. Look for chunky vegetable-based soups and avoid cream-based soups. Most canned soups have a higher GI than soups made from scratch because of the high processing temperatures needed to avoid spoilage. So if you have the time, it is best to make your own. There are a couple of delicious recipes on pages 114 and 120.

BREAKFAST FOODS

Cereals

Many breakfast cereals are high GI. They are made from highly processed grains, which lack both nutrition and fibre. Beware of those so-called healthy granola type of cereals (those that appear to be made up of healthy clusters of grains and nuts), which are usually low in fibre and high in added sugar.

The exceptions are cereals containing at least 10g of fibre per serving. While they are not in themselves much fun, they are easily dressed up into tasty dishes by topping them, for example, with nuts, flaxseed, fruit and Healthy Living Natural Yoghurt.

The king of hot cereals is porridge, made with large flake oats (traditional variety, not instant or quick). It takes about three minutes in the microwave along with toppings such as fruit, sliced almonds/ground flaxseed or fruit yoghurt, and there really is no better way for you and your entire family to start the day.

Cereal bars

Do not be misled by the recent flood of breakfast bars that appear to burst with health. These are high in processed cereals and sugar, and low in fibre. They are not a good choice if you are trying to lose weight. If you are in an unavoidable rush at breakfast time, it's better to go for a Tesco Healthy Living cereal bar with more protein and fibre and less sugar. They are strictly an exception, not the rule. Breakfast is the pivotal meal of the day.

Pancakes/waffles

Packaged pancake mixers and frozen waffles are high GI. However, you can make your own pancakes, crepes and French toast from scratch yourself. See recipes in *Living the Gi Diet* and *The Family Gi Diet* (Virgin Books).

BEVERAGES

See Chapter 3 (page 31).

DAIRY FOODS

Low-fat dairy products are a low GI staple. They are rich in protein, calcium and vitamin D. Full fat dairy foods are not recommended as the fat is mainly saturated (bad) fat. Butter and cheese are amongst the principal villains.

Fruit-flavoured, fat-free yoghurts with a sweetener are ideal for adding to breakfast cereals, as a snack or as a topping on fruit for dessert.

Full-flavoured cheeses such as mature cheddar, feta and Stilton are acceptable in limited quantities as a flavour enhancer; for example, when sprinkled lightly on salads, omelettes and pasta. There is also a a variety of tasty reduced fat cheeses in the Healthy Living range, as well as a heart-healthy cholesterol-reducing cheese, such as Emmicol.

Soya milk is increasingly popular and a good choice if you are lactose intolerant or allergic to dairy products. There are many more gluten-, wheat- and dairy-free products in the Free From Tesco range.

With soya milk look for plain, low-fat versions with added calcium as the flavoured ones can contain high levels of sugar.

BREAD

Interpreting nutritional labelling on breads needs some practice. That healthy-looking seven-grain wholesome loaf may be, on closer inspection, not be what it purports to be. There are two clues: the flour and fibre.

If your seven-grain loaf lists unbleached or enriched white flour as the first ingredient, then most of the bran, fibre and nutrients have been stripped out. The first ingredient should read 100% wholemeal or wholegrain flour. If it is stone-ground, which produces a coarser flour, even better.

Fibre content should be a minimum of 2.5–3g per slice. It's the combination of whole grains with fibre that delivers a lower GI bread.

Other breads that traditionally have been associated with weight loss, such as crispbreads, are low in fibre and have a high GI.

However, the latest high-fibre crispbreads are much more acceptable. Look for at least 2g of fibre per slice.

All bakery products that are made principally from white flour (or 'enriched' flour) including bagels, croissants, baguettes and crumpets are high GI and not recommended if weight control is your concern. Good choices are granary and multigrain bread.

SUMMARY

1. Go shopping mob-handed – taking your children shopping will prove to be a valuable exercise.

2. Clear out the larder of foods on the red list – see page 42.

3. Low GI foods that are low in fat (particularly saturated fat) and sugar are your best choices.

4. Eat lean meat only.

5. The less processed your food is, the better it is for your body.

6. Try to keep to monounsaturated or polyunsaturated fats in your diet.

7. The best breakfast is porridge.

5 Health and reducing the risk of disease

The most alarming medical news about fat, which runs contrary to conventional wisdom, is that it's not (as previously thought) a passive accumulator of energy reserves and extra baggage. Rather it is an active, living part of your body. In fact, it behaves very much like any of our other body organs such as the liver, heart or kidney once it has formed sufficient mass. Excess abdominal fat is now regarded as a root cause for developing cardiovascular abnormalities as well as metabolic complications such as abnormal cholesterol levels, insulin resistance and Type 2 diabetes.

Foods are, in effect, drugs. They have a powerful influence on our health, well-being and emotional state. We take in food four or five times a day, usually with more thought for taste than for nutritional value. It would be incomprehensible to take drugs on the same basis. The right foods can help you maintain your health, extend your life span, give you more energy and make you feel good and sleep better. Couple that with exercise and you are doing all you can to keep healthy, fit and alert. The rest is a matter of genes and luck. Let's take a quick look at the importance of diet, not in fact just managing our weight, but as a critical factor in preventing diseases.

DIABETES

A significant benefit of eating a low GI diet is its impact on people who either suffer from type II diabetes or are at risk of developing the disease. Although this type of diabetes used to predominantly occur in the over-40s, today we are seeing younger and younger people with this disease. The reason it is becoming more predominant in the young is that obese people are far more prone to this type of diabetes and sadly, our teenagers today are increasingly overweight, thanks to their 'couch potato' lifestyle – a bad diet and inactivity.

Type II diabetes stems from the body's inability to utilise insulin to remove excess glucose from the bloodstream. The result is a build-up of glucose in the blood (*hyperglycaemia*), which, if not checked, will ultimately kill the individual.

So control of blood-sugar levels is key to the management of diabetes. That is why a low GI diet is so important for people with type II diabetes and those at risk. Lower GI foods help keep the blood sugars under control by keeping them within the normal range. This helps prevent further complications such as heart disease, stroke, kidney failure and even amputations.

Being overweight and lacking exercise are two of the principal factors that contribute towards diabetes. So, whether you already have diabetes or have been diagnosed at risk, your best chance to minimise medication or avoid it altogether is to lose weight, exercise more and eat a low GI diet. An additional advantage of eating the low GI way is that this will not only help you manage your blood-sugar levels, but it will also help you lose weight. The research evidence is overwhelming.

As there is no cure for diabetes yet, prevention is by far your best option. This is one of the most preventable diseases and you have every opportunity and all the knowledge to do something about it. So get right into your low GI eating and exercise plan and get those pounds off.

Interestingly, more people with diabetes die of heart disease than diabetes, partially because the principal controllable risk factors – being overweight, lacking exercise and bad diet – are all the same. This makes an appropriate bridge to our next disease, heart disease and stroke.

HEART DISEASE AND STROKE

Heart disease and stroke are the cause of 40% of all deaths. It's been calculated that, if we led even a moderate lifestyle (reduced our weight, exercised regularly and quit smoking), we could halve the carnage from these diseases. Though heart disease, like most cancers, is primarily a disease of old age, nearly half of those who suffer heart attacks are under the age of 65.

With regard to diet, the simple fact is that the fatter you are, the more likely it is you will suffer a heart attack or stroke. The two key factors that link heart disease and stroke to diet are hypertension and blood cholesterol.

Hypertension

High blood pressure is the early warning light for both heart disease and stroke. High blood pressure puts more stress on the arterial system and causes it to age and deteriorate more rapidly, ultimately leading to arterial damage, blood clots and heart attack or stroke. Excess weight has a major bearing on high blood pressure.

Cholesterol

Cholesterol is essential to your body's metabolism. However, high blood levels are a problem, as cholesterol is the key ingredient in the plaque that can build up in your arteries, eventually cutting off the blood supply to your heart (causing heart attack) or your brain (leading to stroke). To make things more complicated, there are two forms of cholesterol: HDL (good) cholesterol and LDL (bad) cholesterol. The idea is to boost the HDL level while depressing the LDL level.

Remember it this way: HDL is 'Heart's Delight Level' and LDL is 'Leads to Death Level'!

The villain that raises LDL levels is saturated fat. Conversely, polyunsaturated and monounsaturated fats not only lower LDL levels but also actually boost HDL. The moral: make sure some fat is included in your diet, but make sure it's the right fat. (Refer to Chapter 1 for the complete lowdown on fat.)

CANCER

There is increasing evidence that weight and diet are critical risk factors for most forms of cancer. Diets high in animal fats (saturated), such as some of today's high-protein diets, are directly associated with increased risk of breast, uterine, colon and prostate cancers.

Breast-cancer death rates, for instance, for obese postmenopausal women are 50% higher than for women of normal weight, and obese men are twice as likely to develop colon cancer as men of normal weight.

At a recent meeting of leading cancer researchers, one of the key recommendations for reducing the risk of cancer was that individuals should choose a diet that includes a variety of vegetables, fruits and whole grains – the low GI diet in a nutshell.

ALZHEIMER'S DISEASE

Over the past two to three years there has been a steady flow of research studies all linking Alzheimer's and diet. There appears to be a clear correlation with high saturated fat, which doubles the risk of getting this dreadful disease. Alcohol, salt and high GI carbs are also associated.

On the plus side, a diet rich in deep-sea fish (i.e. oily fish), such as salmon, mackerel and sardines, significantly reduces your risk. It is suggested that omega-3 essential fatty acids and vitamin E found in these fish are the key agents.

The low GI diet, low in saturated fat and rich in omega-3 and vitamin E, is your best defence against Alzheimer's and other dementias.

ARTHRITIS

Yet again, diet appears to have a distinct correlation with managing arthritis and, especially osteoarthritis, in a couple of ways. First, being overweight and/or obese puts a severe strain on joints especially the weight-bearing ones. Knee, hip or ankle may be taking on an extra 22.5–27kg (50–60lb) impact each time your foot hits the ground. Try lifting a 22.5kg (50lb) weight and you'll quickly see what I mean. So get that weight off!

Second, research suggests that eating a diet that is rich in fruit, vegetables, fish (oily fish is the best), nuts, seeds, pulses and whole grains is associated with a reduction in the pain, inflammation and discomfort associated with arthritis – again the low GI diet in a nutshell.

SUMMARY

Eat lower GI foods to help reduce your weight and help:

1. Control blood-sugar levels for management and prevention of diabetes.

2. Lower cholesterol and blood-pressure levels to reduce risk of heart disease and stroke.

3. Reduce saturated fats associated with cancer and Alzheimer's.

4. Reduce inflammation associated with arthritic pain.

6 Getting active with your family

Physical activity isn't just a choice; it's an essential part of your lower GI lifestyle – following a programme of activity can help you to lose more weight while you follow a balanced GI diet, as well as improving your general health and fitness. And getting active with the family is a wonderful way to enjoy some quality time together, even as you're doing yourselves untold good! Exercise need not be daunting. There are so many ways to implement the changes. Rather than slumping in front of the television, get started today.

Take long family walks and breathe in the fresh air. Set aside more time to play with younger kids, veering them away from the television or from computer games. Play with them! Play football, go cycling, go skating, go swimming, fly a kite. Encourage activity-based games such as Twister, hula-hoops and skipping. Go ten-pin bowling or have a round of mini-golf with the little ones. Help your kids find after-school activities that they enjoy by showing them different possibilities. Everyone needs a little inspiration and encouragement. Be there to cheer them on when they're playing football, netball or cricket. Show your partner how proud you are of him when he drags that old squash racquet out of the attic. Plan an activity holiday that all of you can enjoy. There's nothing holding you back but your own imagination!

If you have pets, get active with them too – they'll love the attention and you will all benefit from the exercise involved, e.g. frisbee, ball playing or simply walking the dog. You can also work up a good sweat by getting your cat to run after a piece of string!

WHY GET ACTIVE?

Activity is a good thing in itself – it is essential for good health and for controlling weight.

GOOD NEWS ABOUT ACTIVITY

Facilitates weight loss

Helps keep weight off

Builds muscle tone

Creates a leaner, trimmer body

Makes you feel better

Promotes a 'healthy glow'

Combats tiredness and creates feeling of more energy

Reduces blood fats

Provides a great opportunity for family bonding

How does a GI diet give you a head start with activity?

By choosing lower GI foods you will be getting the majority of your energy from slower-releasing energy foods. So you will be able to go longer without snacking, and feel 'well fuelled' and able to take part in activities after your meals. Always leave at least an hour after eating before doing any activity – 1½–2 hours is ideal. A combination of an apple, banana and a glass of soya milk or semi-skimmed milk 2 hours before is a simple and tasty way to prepare for exercise.

GETTING STARTED

Before you start an exercise programme, do check with your GP. Although they will generally be very supportive, they have details of your medical history and there may be a particular reason why they may want to alter your activity plan. If you have diabetes, do check with your specialist nurse, GP or dietician before you start, as activity will decrease your blood glucose and your insulin needs will be different.

Steps to a fit, active family

1. Start now. It does not have to be complicated to start getting active – start right now; don't put it off until you all have the right trainers, the sky has brightened, you've all lost another couple of pounds, etc. – work out a plan now and commit to it. Seize the day!

2. You are where you are as a family; you're all likely to be at different stages of fitness. It doesn't matter what your starting point is, just begin gently and increase the effort gradually. Remember the tortoise and the hare. It doesn't matter where you have come from; it matters where activity will take you. Today's walk around the park may become a fun-run by the summer and a marathon by next year! The Chinese have a saying for this – 'A journey of a thousand miles starts with a single step.'

3. Do what you enjoy. If walking is the most logical and practical way of the whole family getting some exercise, then walk! If your ambition is to all run round the park without stopping, then walking is a great start. Below are some simple activities to try, and there is a quick guide to activities at the end of this chapter – have a look and you are sure to find something that you enjoy.

- Aim for 30 minutes of moderate activity on at least five days of the week. This may be made up of sessions of a minimum of 10 minutes duration. When you have built up your fitness, the next stage is to aim to complete three sessions of 20 minutes of more intensive activity each week.
- After following an activity plan for three weeks, keep at it, but each week try and go that bit further/faster, etc.
- Try and do some of the above activities at least five times a week for a month.

IDEAS FOR GETTING ACTIVE

Go for a long family walk

Play football

Fly a kite

Buy a skipping rope and do as many jumps as you can in a quarter of an hour

See how far you can swim in half an hour in the local pool

Play mini-golf

Walk the dog

Challenge your partner (and the kids) to a knock-about on the tennis court

Hoover the house

Mow the lawn and do some gardening

Clean the car

Suggest some exciting new after-school activities for the kids

4. Make activity part of your day. Use your imagination to work some form of activity into your daily routine:
- Get off the bus a stop early and walk home.
- Walk the children to school, rather than taking the car.
- Take 30 minutes of your lunch break to walk around outside your workplace at a brisk pace.
- Cycle to work.

5. Choose the right level to exercise at, for you. When you do any activity, focus on working hard enough so that you get slightly out of breath and feel your body warm up. Obviously this will vary depending on the individual. For instance, on a gentle run, you should be able to keep up a conversation at the same time. If you can't talk, you are overdoing it, and if you can recite whole works of Shakespeare, you are not working hard enough!

6. Dress for the part. Active sports involve a modest amount of kit, some of which you may already have, some of which you may need to buy. Make sure each family member is kitted out with the essentials at least. There is a wide selection at Tesco, with many sports items in the Healthy Living range.

SPORTS KIT

A pair of good-quality trainers are invaluable

Loose-fitting activity top and 'bottoms' – ideally with stretchy and 'breathable' fabrics

A water bottle – for every 20 minutes of activity you need to drink 150ml of water, about a third of a pint

---

Race for Life

At Tesco we're always keen to encourage our customers to adopt healthy lifestyles, so we're thrilled once again to be National Sponsor for Cancer Research UK's Race for Life.

Between May and July 2006, there will be over 200 events across the UK. Women of all ages and fitness levels can walk, jog or run the 5km distance to raise vital funds for Cancer Research UK.

To find out more, log on to www.raceforlife.org.

Cancer Research UK 10

For the second year running, Tesco is National Sponsor of the Cancer Research UK 10. These unique fundraising series of 10 kilometre runs are held in the grounds of some of the UK's most beautiful stately homes and are open to both men and women of all running abilities. There will be 5 events in April and a further 30 between September and October.

To register your interest or to join, log on to www.cancerresearchuk10.co.uk.

Tesco Junior & Mini Great Run

Tesco are pleased to sponsor the Junior & Mini Great Runs, the UK's biggest running programme for the Under 17's. The runs are designed to get kids active in a fun and safe environment and an estimated 15,000 children will take part in a series of five races across the country. For more details please visit www.greatrun.org.

Ten ideas for fitness

Different activities can help with the appearance and strength of particular body areas. In order to see real changes you will need to do these activities three times a week, or a combination; for instance, cycle a couple of times to improve your legs and also swim once a week. If you manage 20 minutes duration three times a week the gains will be quicker and you will see the results faster. Ask at your local fitness centre or gym for class details.

ACTIVITY	BENEFIT
1. Running or fast walking	General overall toning
	Weight loss
	Shape up legs
	Benefits the heart and lungs
2. Pilates	Improve saggy stomach muscles
	Control breathing
	Strengthen pelvic floor and lower back
3. Cycling outside or spinning on a static bike	Stamina
	Tone buttock and leg muscles
	Work at your own pace
	Weight loss
	Benefits the heart and lungs
4. Salsa	Tones the waist and hips
	Benefits the heart and lungs
	Fun and social!
5. Yoga	Gentle
	Improves flexibility and posture
	Strengthens muscles
	Promotes relaxation and sleep patterns
6. Swimming	Overall conditioning
	Non-impact – great for starting out/recovering from injury
	Strengthens arms and legs
	Benefits the heart and lungs

7. Trampolining – or mini-rebounder	Improves legs and thighs Benefits the heart and lungs Fun for all the family!
8. Hoovering/gardening/cleaning	Overall moderate intensity workout Strengthens stamina Builds arm muscles Benefits the heart and lungs
9. Skipping	Overall stamina Improves leg muscles Benefits the heart and lungs
10. Frisbee throwing	Gentle overall exercise Improves legs and thighs Stretches muscles Benefits the heart and lungs

SUMMARY

1. Eating lower GI (or slower-releasing energy) foods means that you will be able to go longer without snacking and feel 'well fuelled'.

2. Check with your doctor before embarking on an activity plan.

3. Start your exercise plan slowly, building up as you become more active.

4. Choose exercises that you and your family enjoy doing.

5. Try and do something for twenty minutes three times a week.

7 Eating outside the home

If you wish to manage or lose weight, eating out the low GI way represents one of your biggest challenges. Here you do not have full control over what goes into your meals but you still can make intelligent food choices. In this chapter we'll be dealing with some general guidelines and tips for eating out for all the family. We will be looking specifically at lunch, a time when most of us are eating out of home, fast-food and restaurant dining.

GENERAL GUIDELINES

As dining out is often a social occasion whether it be with family or with friends, it's important that you don't feel that you are a dampener on the occasion and that you are still able to enjoy yourself. Here are a few suggestions:

Eating out

1. Just before you go out, have a small bowl of high-fibre breakfast cereal (such as All-Bran) with skimmed milk or soya milk and sweetener. You could add a couple of spoons of no-fat fruit yoghurt. This will take the edge off your appetite and get some fibre into your stomach, which will help reduce the GI of your upcoming meal.
2. On arrival, order a bottle of mineral water for all the family to drink, instead of letting them drink colas and other sugary soft drinks. A glass of water before your meal will help you feel fuller. A glass of red wine is fine but wait until the main course before drinking.
3. Once the basket of rolls or bread has been passed round, which you should ignore, ask the waiter to remove the basket as the longer it sits there the more tempted you will be to dig in.

4. Order a soup or salad first and tell the waiter you would like this as soon as possible. For soups go for vegetable or bean-based, the chunkier the better. Avoid any that are cream-based. For salads, the golden rule is asking for dressing on the side, as you will only use a fraction of what the restaurant would normally smother on – and avoid salads which come pre-dressed.

5. If you don't have the option of boiled new potatoes or basmati rice, ask for double vegetables instead. We have yet to find a restaurant that won't willingly oblige.

6. Stick with low-fat cuts of meat or poultry where, if necessary, you can remove the skin. Fish and shellfish are an excellent choice but should not be breaded or battered. Remember, as servings tend to be generous in restaurants, eat only 4–6 oz (pack of cards size) and leave the rest.

7. As with salads, ask for any sauces to be put on the side.

8. Desserts. There are not usually a lot of low GI choices. Fresh fruit and berries, if available, are your best choice without the ice cream. Most other choices are a dietary disaster. The best advice is to try and avoid dessert. Have a low GI starter and main course instead. However if you do have a dessert then ask for extra forks so it can be shared!

9. Only order decaffeinated coffee. Skimmed decaf cappuccino is our family's favourite choice. Avoid liqueurs and hot chocolate.

10. Finally and perhaps most importantly, eat slowly. Try putting your fork down between mouthfuls.

The stomach can take between 20 and 30 minutes to let the brain know it feels full. So if you eat quickly, you may be shovelling in more food than you require till the brain says stop. You will also have more time to savour your meal.

WHAT TO HAVE FOR LUNCH

Since most of us spend the lunch hour away from home, either at work, college or school, we tend to have two options for the midday meal:
• take our own, or
• eat at a restaurant.
In both cases, eating the low GI way is definitely doable – but there are some important guidelines to keep in mind.

Bring your own

This is really the best option for the GI dieter. When you pack your own lunch, you can be sure that all the ingredients used are low GI. And as far as the kids go, it's a good way to keep an eye on what they are eating throughout the day. If children are given the opportunity to try healthy, fresh alternatives to the stodgy, processed convenience food they're used to eating, they will blossom. Contrary to popular belief, kids are not genetically programmed to exist on a diet of burgers and chips! Show them the way forward and they will respond fantastically well.

Here are some tips for turning a regular packed lunch into a low GI one. Also, take a look at the recipes at the end of this book (for example, Spinach salad with lentils and feta, Turkey wrap and fruity rice salad) for some mouth-watering suggestions for packed lunches that everyone can enjoy.

• **Sandwiches.** Watch out for the high GI and high calorie ones. There are several things you can do to make your sandwich low GI. First, use one slice of 100% stone-ground wholemeal or other high fibre bread. Spread on some mustard or hummus (no mayonnaise, butter or margarine) and top with 115g (4oz) of lean deli ham, chicken, turkey or fish. Add at least three vegetables, such as lettuce, tomato, onion or green pepper, and do not top the sandwich with another slice of bread – simply eat it open-faced. Avoid egg, chicken and tuna salad sandwiches that are made with high calorie mayonnaise.

- **Salads**. Salads are almost always low GI but are often short on protein. Add in chickpeas or other types of beans, tuna, salmon, tofu or 115g (4oz) of skinless, cooked chicken breast or other lean meat. Also watch the dressing. Use only low-fat or fat-free versions.
- **Soups**. In general, commercially canned soups have a relatively high GI rating because of the necessary high temperatures used in the canning process. Homemade soups made with low GI ingredients are the best option. Beware of all cream-based or puréed vegetable soups, since they are high in fat and heavily processed.
- **Pasta**. The thing to watch out for here is quantity. Your pasta dish should contain only 40g (1½oz) pasta (dry weight), with lots of vegetables, light pasta sauce and 115g (4oz) of chicken or lean deli meat. But this still leaves you with dozens of delicious combinations.
- **Cottage cheese, fruit and nuts**. A fast and easy lunch to take to work is cottage cheese mixed with fruit and sliced almonds.
- **Dessert**. Always have some fresh fruit for dessert.

Lunching out

SIT-DOWN RESTAURANTS

All you have to do is order a meal that includes a low-fat source of protein, such as chicken or fish, and vegetables. Ask for extra vegetables in place of potatoes or rice, since restaurants tend to serve the high GI versions. For other general dining-out suggestions see the first section in this chapter.

ALL-YOU-CAN-EAT BUFFETS

These can be your best or worst choice depending on your self-control – best, because you're free to make your own selection and there are usually lots of options for a low GI plate; worst, because it's tempting to have a little bit of everything and then wish you'd taken a larger plate! If you're anything like us, by the time you are half way round the buffet table, your plate is already full and you try to pile on those tantalising foods that you wished you had seen earlier. The secret is to do a quick survey of the whole buffet before picking up your plate and starting. Just follow the low GI ground rules: have a look at all the options first and the buffet will definitely be your best dining-out option.

INTERNATIONAL CUISINE

We love trying new foods from different countries. It is a huge subject in its own right and space limitations here unfortunately do not allow for detailed recommendations.

From a low GI standpoint your best choices are Italian, as long as you watch your serving sizes of pasta, although pizza is a definite no-no. Otherwise apply the general green-light rule when choosing food and use your common sense.

FAST FOOD

Fast-food chains

For most of us fast food is a convenient and popular choice but it is full of pitfalls unless you're very wary. Let the following be your guide.

Up until recently it would have been really difficult to get a green-light meal at a fast-food restaurant. However, the major fast-food chains are now offering some healthy options.

- Salads, usually with grilled chicken, are your best choice.
- Always ask for low-fat dressings.
- Drink water instead of cola or other fizzy drinks.

Other fast food

Fast food-wise there is not much else better on offer. Sandwich shops are little better. We suggest that you check the menus at all fast-food outlets to see whether healthy low-GI food is on offer. If it isn't, say why you are not buying anything – the more the customer asks or complains, the more likely the outlet is to change.

Because of our need for value for money, convenience and speed, we all use take-away outlets, but considerable caution is required. Nutrition should be our first thought, not convenience.

FISH AND CHIPS

Fish and chips is the UK's best-known take-away food. However, fish and chips eaten on a regular basis can lead to obesity – they are a classic example of taking an ideal food, fish, adulterating it with calorie-loaded batter and deep-frying it in oil. Once you add the deep-fried potatoes, healthy nutrition is the last thing on your mind!

CHINESE

In the main Chinese dishes are not a good choice, but if you choose carefully and avoid the obvious pitfalls such as glutinous rice and sweet sauces you can usually find some dishes on the menu to suit. Steamed vegetables are the best area to aim for. You will find high sodium levels in many of the sauces and most restaurants use saturated oils in cooking. There are better options for take-away so use them infrequently.

INDIAN

Indian cuisine uses a lot of fruit, vegetables, legumes and whole grains, which is the good news. On the other hand, Indian food is typically high in fat. Keep away from food that has been cooked with 'ghee' (clarified and evaporated butter), a highly saturated fat which is frequently used. Choose baked or grilled dishes such as Tandoori instead of those covered in thick sauces.

PARTY FOOD

If you're going to a party, beware the canapés; party finger food is tempting, but usually very fattening. Eat something before you arrive and go for vegetables, fruit, crudités dipped in hummus or low-fat dip if available. Never drink alcohol on an empty stomach – and remember to drink lots of mineral water. If throwing a children's party, take inspiration from some of the many GI recipes available; for example, Turkey wraps, Nutty banana sandwiches made with wholemeal bread, Ricotta cake, Peach and raspberry cups or Pesto pitta pockets will make delicious, healthy alternatives to the usual party fare.

WHAT TO SNACK ON

It can't be stressed enough how important it is to have three snacks every day. Snacks play a critical role between meals by giving you a boost when you most need it. Choose fruit, fat-free fruit yoghurt with sweetener, cottage cheese, raw vegetables or nuts. Watch out for other products that claim to be fat- and sugar-free, such as packaged puddings. Unfortunately these products are usually made with highly processed grain and are high GI.

You might also want to look into nutrition (cereal) bars. Choose 50–65g bars that have around 200 calories each with 20–30g of carbohydrates, 12–15g of protein and 5g of fat – Tesco Healthy Living nutrition bars are a good choice. The rest are often high GI, high calorie, and contain lots of quick-fix carbs. Check the labels carefully.

SUMMARY

Remember when eating out:

1. Bowl of bran cereal before going out.

2. Drink water on arrival – red wine later with the main course.

3. Ask for the bread basket to be taken away from the table.

4. Choose a soup or salad for the first course, preferably a vegetable/bean soup and not cream-based. Ask for salad dressings to be served separately.

5. Two vegetables in lieu of potatoes/rice.

6. Poultry, veal and seafood are the best choices for the main course. Never choose fried food.

7. All sauces should be served on the side.

8. Desserts: avoid, or ask for extra forks to share. Choose fresh fruit/berries, if available.

9. Choose decaffeinated coffee; avoid liqueurs and hot chocolate.

10. Eat slowly.

8 Your GI questions and answers

Remember to consult your doctor prior to starting any diet or activity plan. Reading this book may have raised some queries and here are some of the most common questions that we get.

Q: Is the GI Diet just for people who want to lose weight?
A: No, it is for people who want to maintain or control their current weight as well as for those who want to lose a few pounds – or even for people just wanting to eat more healthily and feel better.

Q: Can I eat unlimited lower GI food?
A: No. Since some lower GI foods are high in calories and saturated fat they should be avoided (see listings on page 129 for your best choices). Otherwise moderation and common sense are your best guides.

Q: Is the GI Diet suitable for children?
A: Yes. The GI Diet with its emphasis on fruits, vegetables, whole grains, nuts, lean meat/fish and low-fat dairy is ideal for building and nourishing young bodies from the age of five. It also helps establish healthy eating patterns that will live with them throughout their adult life. Remember that growing children need sufficient fat in their diet – the good kind of fat, found in fish, nuts and vegetable oils.

Q: How do I integrate the GI Diet into family life?
A: The good thing about GI is that you won't need to hammer the point home – by subtly adapting many of your family's usual recipes you will already be on the way to a new eating lifestyle. Firstly, though, empty your larder and fridge of high GI undesirables such as white bread, cakes and sweets, leaving you free to start with a clean

slate. This will also give your family a clear message that things are about to change for the better – but with the minimum of fuss! Also, with the GI Diet, there is no need to sacrifice taste or convenience for the sake of keeping within the GI guidelines. There are countless delicious GI recipes to help enrich family mealtimes.

Q: I want to throw a birthday party for my little girl who's turning four. What can I lay on, food-wise, that will please all her friends as well as being GI-friendly? I don't want to undo all our good work, but I want to keep all concerned happy!

A: Why not get inspired by some of the many GI recipes available? Nutty banana sandwiches, Ricotta cake, Peach and raspberry cups or Pesto pitta pockets make delicious, healthy alternatives to the usual party fare. When making sandwiches, always go for wholegrain bread. Fill with hummus, cucumber, low-fat cheese and tomato or deli ham. Lay on lots of raw vegetables to snack on, sparkly water with lemon and water, maybe some watered down reduced-sugar juices. Make your own birthday cake using lots of strawberries. If the kids enjoy the odd piece of high-cocoa chocolate (such as Tesco Finest 72% cocoa), it isn't the end of the world! The good thing about the GI way of eating is that it offers plenty of flexibility and plenty of options for all members of the family.

Q: My thirteen-year-old son is very unadventurous when it comes to food. His eating habits seem to consist of pasta, pasta and pasta, broken up with the odd pizza. What can I do to broaden his horizons?

A: Teenage boys can be a law unto themselves! There's nothing wrong with pasta, particularly if your son sticks to tomato-based sauces rather than cream-based ones which are unnecessarily high in fat. Try making your own pasta sauces, crammed full of fresh ingredients, and freeze a load so you are well prepared in advance.

Try incorporating mushrooms, peppers, courgettes, carrots, artichoke hearts, olives, fresh herbs, capers into your pasta sauce ... the list is endless! Just be sure to serve a huge, delicious salad on the side and continue serving up a good variety of different healthy dishes to the rest of the family. One day your son might surprise you.

Q. My sixteen-year-old daughter is obsessed with the way she looks – her hair, her skin, her clothes and, of course, her figure. I've just started the whole family on the GI Diet but I'm worried that all this talk about diets will lead to her developing an eating disorder.
A. It's true that obsessing about dieting can be damaging. Your own behaviour as a role model will have the greatest impact on your child's relationship with food, so it's up to you to have a healthy, moderate relationship with food. But there is nothing obsessive about the GI Diet. In many ways the word "diet" is unfortunate as it has become associated with weight loss rather than just a way of eating. The GI Diet is intended to be the way you will eat the rest of your life; a healthy, active and long one. Rest assured that, rather than becoming over-preoccupied with calorie counting and weighing herself, your daughter will be delighted with the results of eating the GI way – and she'll love the healthy glow it gives her skin, too!

Q. Can I use the GI Diet if I am pregnant or breastfeeding?
A. The GI Diet is ideal for pregnancy and while breastfeeding. In both cases, make sure you are taking three to four servings daily of low-fat dairy products such as skimmed milk. Additionally, when pregnant you should ensure you are getting sufficient prenatal nutrients such as folic acid and iron. Though most of these are present in the GI Diet, your health care provider will probably recommend a supplement. Often it is recommended you have a vitamin supplement to ensure

you are getting sufficient key vitamins such as C and B Complex. But supplements containing vitamin A should only be taken under medical supervision. In all cases, make sure you discuss your change in diet with your health professional before you start.

Q. I have elderly parents coming to dinner at the weekend – can I feed them a GI meal?
A. Of course. There is nothing harmful about the GI way of eating, and if you follow some of our specially devised GI recipes, your parents will thoroughly enjoy their meal and may not even notice it is based on the GI Diet.

Q. My husband won't hear of a diet – how can I convince him of coming on board?
A. GI is more than just a diet – it's a way of life. And as such, there's no need to terrorise your husband with the thought of all the tasty food he will be missing out on if he follows it. Either concentrate on your own GI plan and let your husband follow by example when he sees the new, slim-line, healthy you – or subtly adjust the menu along GI guidelines without making a big deal about it. Before he knows it, your husband will be well on the way to a GI lifestyle and wondering where all his surplus weight went!

Q: Can I just follow the GI plan without getting more active?
A: Yes, but if you want to lose weight your weight loss won't be as fast as it would if you exercise. Also, you won't have the fitness gains and enjoy the 'feel good' factor that comes with it; you will miss out on the extra body definition that comes with muscle gain. This in turn will mean that you won't increase your metabolism and thus burn more calories each day.

Q: What are the guidelines for good health?
A: A balanced diet is made up of a mix of foods from the four main food groups:
• bread, other cereals and potatoes
• fruit and vegetables
• meat, fish and alternatives
• milk and dairy foods.
Foods containing fat or sugar can also be incorporated into a healthy diet, but these should be in smaller amounts. Follow the Government's '8 tips for healthy eating', as below:
• Base your meal on starchy foods
• Eat a lot of fruit and vegetables
• Eat more fish
• Cut down on saturated fat and sugar
• Try to eat less salt – no more than 6g a day
• Get active and try to be a healthy weight
• Drink plenty of water
• Don't skip breakfast

Q: What about alcohol? I like a drink every now and then.
A: Alcohol should be avoided if you hope to lose weight. If, however, you have reached your target weight, a maximum of one glass of wine with dinner is allowed. (See page 32 for more information.)

Q: How much water should I drink?
A: About 2 litres a day – this is 8–10 cups or glasses (200ml) a day. One tip is to take a large bottle of water to work and aim to finish it by the end of the day. Water is an essential part of getting and staying healthy. Over half of the body consists of water. Water is continuously lost from our bodies during the day through urine, sweat and even in our breath. It is important to keep a check on our

water (hydration) levels and replace lost fluids. Even a small reduction in hydration can have a direct impact on our long-term health – it can also reduce our concentration span and stop us exercising or playing sport as well as we would want to. Remember, thirst is a poor indicator of dehydration. Drink regularly before you feel thirsty.

Q: I have 'fallen off the wagon'. How do I get back on it?
A: It is normal to experience the odd lapse in following a dietary plan and it is all part of the process of changing from one way of eating to another. Don't beat yourself up about it. Decide to move on and concentrate on the future. Simply start where you left off, with renewed confidence. (See page 23.)

Q: Will the GI Diet work for vegetarians?
A: Yes. The GI Diet is all about carbohydrate-containing foods, which are equally acceptable to vegetarians. The protein part of the meal, such as the meat, poultry, fish or eggs, can be swapped for other sources of protein, such as soya, mycoprotein (e.g. Quorn), nuts, seeds, pulses or dairy products. Some of these, such as nuts and pulses, have the added advantage of having a lower GI themselves.

Q: Is skipping meals or snacks a problem?
A: Yes. Missing meals is not going to help you achieve a healthier, more energetic you. Breakfast is the most important meal of the day as it kick-starts your metabolism and gives you energy plus important vitamins and minerals. If you don't eat breakfast, it is more difficult to make up your requirement for vitamins and minerals later in the day and you may overcompensate with high GI foods. Eating regularly will help to stabilise your blood sugar levels and help you to feel fuller for longer. It will also prevent dips in energy throughout the day.

Q: What should I look for in food labels?

A: Look out for the blue 'low' and 'medium' GI circle on the front of Tesco own-brand products and check out the website for a complete list of tested lower GI foods. These foods have been fully tested and been found to be lower GI. Only foods containing carbohydrate can be tested for GI, e.g. breads, pasta, rice, ready-made meals, cereals, pulses, fruit and vegetables, as it is a measure of the effect of starches and sugars on the blood sugar. You won't therefore find the GI circle on foods containing very low or no carbs, such as meat, poultry, fish, dairy products etc.

Guideline Daily Amounts (GDAs) appear on the back of many Tesco-branded products and give an indication of the contribution a serving of a product makes towards your daily recommended intake of calories, fat and salt. For more information on label contents see page 32.

Q: I am gluten intolerant. Can I still use the GI Diet?

A: Yes, absolutely, as long as the foods you choose are free of gluten (found in wheat, barley, rye and oats). There are now many gluten-free alternatives to ordinary foods on the market. Tesco stocks an excellent range of Free From foods, and has a total of 170 different products that are gluten- and wheat-free. Many of these are lower GI. The Gluten-free diet plan, available at www.tescodiets.com, will help you follow a healthy and varied diet while avoiding all sources of gluten and is suitable for people with Coeliac disease.

Q: How do I remember the GI ratings for each food?
A: Tesco is making this easy for customers by starting a programme of food labelling – so look for the blue label. You don't need to remember numbers themselves, just general foods that are lower GI, such as basmati rice or granary bread – a few simple changes will add up to something powerful. Information on the Tesco GI online diet plan is available at www.tescodiets.com. You will also find information published in store.

Q: Will I still be able to go out to restaurants?
A: Of course! Try to remember a few key foods that are lower GI, such as granary breads, basmati rice, pasta, and most fruits and vegetables. Base your meal choices around these and this will bring down the overall GI value of the meal. If you have difficulty in finding these choices on the menu, ask the manager if they'll consider providing some in the future. Remember restaurants like to supply what their clientele demands! Here are some pointers:
• Italian – pasta, mixed salads (choose low-fat dressings such as yoghurt-based ones)
• Indian – basmati rice (check with the restaurant), noodles and dishes containing pulses such as dhal
• Chinese – avoid, but, if you do eat this type of food, choose noodles or dishes containing nuts or beans/peas
• English – pasta, noodles, small new potatoes, beans, peas, lentils, granary bread, fruit and vegetables.

9 Menu plans and recipes

In order to get you started, we have composed menu plans for seven days' worth of meals. Hopefully, they'll show you just how broad a variety of foods you can eat and how tasty recipes with lower GI foods can be. These recipes are not necessarily appropriate for those concerned with weight loss – they represent an across-the-board selection of healthy meals for you and all the family to enjoy, in fact there's plenty to keep the kids rushing to the dinner table. In many cases you can substitute some ingredients with low-fat equivalents. All the ingredients should be available at your local Tesco. Bon appetit!

Recipes that are suitable for weight loss are marked with a ✪

DAY 1:

Breakfast

100g Tesco Healthy Living baked beans with 2 slices of Tesco Multigrain Batch Loaf (50g each) and a small glass of unsweetened fruit juice. 1 serving of a fruit of choice.

Lunch

Turkey sandwich with cranberry sauce: Fill 2 slices of Tesco Multigrain Batch Loaf (50g each) with 50g turkey slices, 2 tsp cranberry sauce and 25g Tesco Healthy Living Coleslaw. 1 pear.

Dinner

Tuna spaghetti with chunky tomatoes, lemon and basil (see page 110)

DAY 2:

Breakfast

Tesco Fruit Muesli (50g) with 125ml semi-skimmed milk. Tesco low fat yoghurt. 1 Mandarin, Satsuma or Clementine.

Lunch

Pitta with hummus and salad: Fill a Tesco wholemeal pitta bread with 75g hummus, 25g lower fat cheese, a sliced tomato, a handful of mixed salad leaves and 6 black olives. Tesco Healthy Living light yoghurt.

Dinner

Vegetable and chicken skewers (see page 100)

DAY 3:

Breakfast

Measure out 25g Tesco porridge oats and add three times the volume of semi-skimmed milk. Cook following package directions. Top with stewed apple or rhubarb. 1 banana.

Lunch

Chicken Salad Sandwich with Mustard Mayonnaise: Spread 2 slices of Tesco Finest Crusty Malted Wheat Bread with a mixture of 1 tsp of reduced fat mayonnaise and mustard to taste. Fill with 100g chicken fillet and top with rocket.

Dinner

Salmon Teriyaki with sesame noodles (see page 110)

DAY 4:

Breakfast

Scrambled egg on a slice of Tesco Multigrain Batch Loaf (50g slice) with 2 grilled tomatoes. Tesco Probiotic yoghurt.

Lunch

Middle Eastern Pasta Salad: Cook 75g Tesco dried pasta according to package directions, omitting any suggested fat or salt. In a blender, combine 50g chickpeas, canned and drained, a squeeze of lemon juice, a small clove of garlic, a tsp soy sauce and a tbs chopped fresh parsley. Blend to a paste and mix into the cooked pasta, along with a tbs each of chopped red onion and red pepper.

Dinner

Red chicken with Cuban rice (see page 101)

DAY 5:

Breakfast

2 slices of Tesco organic malt loaf with a banana

Lunch

Tuna Pitta: Mix 100g tuna, canned in brine and drained, with 1 tbs of lower fat mayonnaise. Use to fill a Tesco wholegrain pitta bread and top with plenty of salad.

Dinner

Veggie Chilli Con Carne (see page 121)

DAY 6:

Breakfast

50g Tesco Fruit n Nut Muesli with 100ml semi-skimmed milk. 1 Tesco Probiotic Yoghurt.

Lunch

Tuna & Sweetcorn Sandwich: Mix 50g tuna with a tbs lower fat mayonnaise and 50g Tesco no added salt or sugar sweetcorn. Use to fill 2 slices of Tesco Multigrain Batch Loaf (50g each) and top with mixed salad leaves.

Dinner

Thai-style pork and vegetable stir-fry (see page 92)

DAY 7:

Breakfast

Greek Yoghurt with muesli and fruit: 3 tbs of lower fat Greek style yoghurt with tbs Tesco Wholewheat muesli. 2 plums.

Lunch

Ham or Turkey Salad Sandwich: Mix a tsp reduced fat mayonnaise with mustard to taste and spread over 2 slices of Tesco Multigrain Batch Loaf (50g each). Fill with 2 slices of roast ham or turkey and salad. 2 plums.

Dinner

Spice-crusted tuna with cherry tomato compote (see page 113)

MEAT

CRISPY BACON AND MUSHROOM SALAD

SERVES 2

3 streaky bacon rashers
2 tbsp olive oil
2 tsp Dijon mustard
1 garlic clove, crushed

salt and black pepper
75g (3oz) mixed salad leaves
75g (3oz) chestnut mushrooms, thinly sliced

1. Preheat the grill and cook the bacon until crisp and golden. Cool and break each rasher into three pieces.
2. Meanwhile make the dressing by whisking the olive oil, a little at a time, into the mustard. If the dressing is very thick, loosen it with a few drops of hot water. Stir in the garlic and season with salt and freshly ground black pepper.
3. Just before serving, toss the salad leaves, bacon and mushrooms together and drizzle with the dressing.

WARM EGG AND BACON SALAD

SERVES 4

6 large organic eggs
1 x 200g pack back bacon, cut into strips, or 1 x 200g pack bacon bits
1 x 225g pack baby spinach
1 x pack romaine lettuce hearts, washed and torn into bite-sized pieces
1 x 250g pack cherry tomatoes, halved
6–8 tbsp of your favourite salad dressing

1. Hard-boil and quarter or roughly chop the eggs.
2. Fry the bacon in a non-stick pan until crisp and golden.
3. Combine the spinach, the romaine lettuce hearts and the tomatoes in a bowl.
4. Toss the salad with the salad dressing and top with the eggs and bacon. Serve with crusty wholegrain or multigrain baguette, if wished.

HAM, CHEESE AND BLACK OLIVE PIZZAS

SERVES 4

2 cloves garlic, crushed
2 tbsp olive oil
4 pitta breads
200g (7oz) grated mozzarella
200g (7oz) smoked ham, cut into strips
50g (1¾ oz) pitted black olives, sliced
salt and black pepper
½ x 20g pack fresh basil, roughly torn

1. Preheat the grill. Stir the garlic into the olive oil. Open up the pitta breads to make eight 'pizza' bases. Lay them on two separate baking sheets and scatter with the grated mozzarella.

2. Top the pizzas with ham and black olives, then drizzle with the garlic oil. Season with salt and freshly ground black pepper and grill half the pizzas for 4–5 minutes, until the base is crisp and the topping is oozing and golden. Top with the basil and serve. Cook the second batch as you tuck in.

PORK WITH A ROSEMARY, APRICOT AND BACON STUFFING

SERVES 6

for the stuffing:
15g (½ oz) butter
1 onion, finely chopped
1 x 200g pack bacon bits
150g (5½oz) dried ready-to-eat apricots, roughly chopped
½ tbsp chopped fresh rosemary
salt and freshly ground black pepper

for the pork:
1 x 1.5kg (3lb 5oz) boneless loin or shoulder of pork
1 tsp salt
½ tbsp vegetable oil

1. Preheat the oven to 220°C, 425°F, Gas 7. First, make the stuffing. Melt the butter in a frying pan over low heat. Cook the onions and bacon for 10 minutes until softened. Remove from the heat, stir in the apricots and rosemary. Season with salt and pepper. Allow the stuffing to cool.

2. Place the pork on a board, skin side up, and score the rind at 2.5cm (1in) intervals. The easiest way to do this is by using a Stanley knife. Turn the meat skin side down and place the cooled stuffing down the middle. Roll up the pork and tie very tightly with string. Rub the skin with salt and oil and roast for 25 minutes.

3. Lower the heat to 190°C, 375°F, Gas 5 and cook for 1 hour 5 minutes (or 20 minutes per 450g/1lb), until it is cooked right through. Rest the meat for 10 minutes before serving.

WARM SAUSAGE, SPINACH AND CANNELLINI BEAN SALAD

SERVES 4

4 pork sausages
3 tbsp olive oil
2 garlic cloves, crushed
2 x 300g tins cannellini beans
1 small red onion, thinly sliced
100g (3½oz) baby spinach
zest and juice of 1 lemon
salt and black pepper

1. Preheat the grill. Place the sausages on a roasting sheet and put under the grill for 5 minutes on each side, until cooked through and golden. Cut into thick slices.

2. Meanwhile, put the olive oil and garlic in a wide saucepan and heat gently for 1 minute. Stir in the cannellini beans and sliced onion. Season with salt and freshly ground black pepper and continue to cook over a low heat for 5 minutes to soften.

3. Remove the pan from the heat and toss in the sausages, along with the spinach, and lemon zest and juice.

4. Transfer to a large salad bowl and season with salt and pepper.

BEEF THAI RED CURRY WITH NOODLES

SERVES 4

175g (6oz) egg noodles
1 tbsp vegetable oil
600g (1lb 5oz) sirloin steak, trimmed of fat and sliced 1cm (½in) thick
90g pot red Thai curry paste
1 x 400g can coconut milk
1 tbsp honey
2.5cm (1in) piece ginger, peeled and thickly sliced
1 lemon-grass stalk, bashed (optional)
100g (3½ oz) mangetout, sliced diagonally
3 tbsp fish sauce (Nam pla) or salt to taste
zest of a lime
small handful of fresh coriander leaves

1. Cook the noodles in a large pan of boiling water as per packet directions. Drain and set aside.
2. Meanwhile, heat the oil in a casserole dish over a high heat and add the steak and curry paste, stirring to coat the beef. Cook on all sides for about a minute, until lightly golden, but still pink in the middle. Pour in the coconut milk and all the remaining ingredients, except the coriander. Bring to the boil and cook for two minutes further, until the mangetout are tender.
3. Remove the ginger and lemon grass (if using). Toss the curry with the noodles and top with the coriander.

PAN-FRIED VENISON MEDALLION WITH RED CABBAGE CONFIT ⭐

SERVES 4

40g (1½ oz) unsalted butter
2 tbsp olive oil
500g (1lb 2oz) red cabbage, finely shredded
1 x 75cl bottle red wine
50g (1¾oz) cooked natural beetroot, grated
2 x 280g packs venison steaks
15g (½oz) coarsely ground peppercorns
3 tbsp shallots, finely chopped
4 tbsp *Finest* beef stock
salt

1. Melt 25g (1oz) of butter in a saucepan with 1 tbsp oil. Cook the red cabbage for 4–5 minutes, stirring occasionally, then add the wine and beetroot and simmer for 45–50 minutes until tender and about 100ml (3½fl oz) of liquid is left in the pan.

2. Coat the venison steaks in the pepper and sprinkle with a little salt. Set to one side.

3. Melt 15g (½oz) of butter and 1 tbsp oil in a frying pan over medium high heat and cook steaks for about 5 minutes each side for medium rare. Allow 2–3 minutes longer on each side for well done. Cover the pan and allow the meat to rest.

4. Add the shallots to the pan used to cook the meat and cook for two minutes. Strain the liquid from the cabbage and add the stock. Simmer and reduce by half.

5. To serve, place a steak on the plate, spoon the cabbage round and finish with the sauce.

PASTA WITH LAMB SAUCE

SERVES 4

300g (10½oz) lamb steaks
10 fresh rosemary sprigs
1 onion, sliced
4–5 tbsp extra virgin olive oil
175ml (6fl oz) dry white wine
1 x 400g can tomatoes, chopped
400g (14oz) pappardelle
salt and freshly ground black pepper
5 tbsp freshly grated Parmesan to serve

1. Rinse the lamb steaks and pat them dry with kitchen paper, then cut them carefully into uniform-sized cubes.
2. Chop the rosemary and sliced onion together. In a saucepan over a medium heat, fry the rosemary and onion in the olive oil until the onion is soft and clear but not browned. Add the meat and brown it thoroughly on all sides. Pour in the wine and boil for about 2 minutes to boil off the alcohol, then add the tomatoes and stir. Season, then simmer very gently for about 1½ hours.
3. When the sauce is ready, cook the pasta according to pack instructions. Drain it carefully and return to the saucepan. Pour over the lamb sauce and toss to incorporate. Transfer to warm bowls, sprinkle with cheese and serve.

THAI-STYLE PORK AND VEGETABLE STIR-FRY

SERVES 4

1 tbsp groundnut oil
250g (9oz) pork mince
3 tbsp red Thai curry paste
1 large red onion, halved and sliced
2 large carrots, grated
1 large courgette, shredded
125g (4½oz) green cabbage, shredded
1–2 tbsp water or chicken stock
lime wedges, torn basil leaves and roasted peanuts (if wished) to garnish

1. Heat the oil in a wok or large frying pan and brown the pork mince. Stir in the red Thai curry paste (a little extra may be added if desired).
2. Add the onion, carrots, courgette and cabbage. Stir-fry for 1–2 minutes, adding the water or chicken stock to moisten.
3. Top with the basil leaves, lime wedges and roasted peanuts, if wished. Serve with freshly cooked Thai noodles.

POTATO SALAD WITH GREEN BEANS, FETA AND CHORIZO

SERVES 4

500g (1lb 2oz) new potatoes
1 x 250g pack green beans
1 x 250g pack cherry tomatoes, halved
1 x 200g pack feta cheese, crumbled
1 x 20g pack flat leaf parsley, chopped
125g (4½oz) chorizo, sliced
1 tbsp wine vinegar
crisp salad leaves to serve

1. In separate saucepans, cook the potatoes and the green beans in boiling salted water until just tender, then drain.
2. Once the potatoes are cool enough to handle, cut them in half and place in a bowl with the green beans, tomatoes, feta and parsley and set aside.
3. Dry-fry the chorizo. Add it and all its oil from the pan to the bowl along with the wine vinegar.
4. Serve with crisp salad leaves.

MOUSSAKA BAKED IN AUBERGINES ⭐

SERVES 4

2 very large aubergines, each weighing about 400g (14oz),
or 4 x 200g (7oz) aubergines
1 tbsp salt
1 tbsp olive oil
1 onion, chopped
1 x 500g pack lean steak mince
2 garlic cloves, finely chopped
½ tsp ground cinnamon
1 tbsp dried oregano
2 tbsp tomato puree
½ tsp honey or sugar
2 tbsp chopped fresh parsley
1 x 300g tub *Finest* beef stock
Freshly ground black pepper
for the topping:
15g (½oz) butter
15g (½oz) plain flour
150ml (¼pt) milk
150ml (¼pt) Greek-style yogurt
1 egg yolk

1. Cut the aubergines in half and scrape out most of the flesh leaving a wall about 5mm (¼in) thick all the way round. Sprinkle with the salt and set aside. Chop the flesh.

2. To make the stuffing, heat the oil and sauté the onion and aubergine flesh. Add the mince and garlic and cook until well browned. Add the remaining ingredients, cover and simmer for 45 minutes.

3. Preheat the oven to 190°C/ 375°F/Gas 5. Rinse and dry the aubergine shells and set them in a baking dish. Fill with the mince and cook for 45 minutes.

4. Meanwhile, make the white sauce with the butter, flour and milk. Simmer for 1 minute until thickened and smooth. Remove from the heat, whisk in the yogurt and egg yolk. Spoon over the aubergines and return to the oven for 15 minutes. Drizzle over any cooking juices and serve with a spinach salad and new potatoes if wished.

MODERN IRISH STEW

SERVES 4-6

2 x packs British lamb chops (5–7 chops per pack)
1 x 500g pack baby onions
750g baby new potatoes
1 x 270g pack mini carrots
few sprigs lemon thyme
2 tbsp plain flour
600ml (1pt) lamb stock
salt and freshly ground black pepper
chopped parsley and chives to garnish

1. Preheat oven to 180°C, 350°F, Gas 4. Brown the chops in a non-stick frying pan, then layer up in a large flameproof casserole with the vegetables and thyme, seasoning between layers.
2. Pour off the excess fat from the frying pan and add the flour. Stir well to make a paste, then cook for 30 seconds. Stir in the stock to make a smooth sauce and bring to the boil.
3. Pour the liquid over the meat and vegetables and bring to a simmer on the hob. Cover and cook in the lower half of the oven for 2 hours or until the lamb is tender. Garnish with the freshly chopped herbs and serve with Savoy cabbage, if wished.

MARINATED LAMB STEAKS WITH SWEET POTATO MASH

SERVES 4-6

1 tbsp clear honey
zest and juice of 1 orange
1 tbsp chopped mint
1–2 garlic cloves, crushed
salt and pepper
2 x 500g packs lamb leg steaks
1kg (2lb 4oz) sweet potatoes
knob of butter (optional)
4 tbsp water or stock
chopped mint to garnish

1. Combine the honey, orange zest and juice, mint and garlic. Season generously.
2. Pour the marinade over the lamb steaks, cover and leave to marinate for 1 hour or up to 24 hours in the fridge, turning occasionally.
3. For the mash, steam or cook the sweet potatoes in boiling water for about 20 minutes, drain and mash with a knob of butter if desired and season.
4. Drain the steaks, reserving the marinade, and fry or grill over/under a medium heat until crisp and golden – about 15 minutes.
5. Add the reserved marinade and the water or stock to the frying pan or bubble separately to make a sauce. Spoon over the chops and serve with the mash, garnished with the mint.

SPRING LAMB WITH PEAS, MINT AND LITTLE GEMS

SERVES 4-6

1 leg of British spring lamb, weighing about 1.8kg (4lb), boned (keep the bone) and excess fat removed, cut in 2.5–4cm (1–1.5in) pieces; or use about 1kg (2lb 4oz) diced lean lamb
2 tbsp vegetable oil
2 medium carrots, peeled and quartered
2 medium onions, halved through the root
1 stick celery, quartered

1 leek, trimmed, rinsed and quartered
6 garlic cloves
50g (1¾oz) butter
2 bay leaves
1 sprig thyme
2 tsp tomato puree
1 tbsp plain flour
½ bottle dry white wine
300ml (½pt) lamb stock or water
250g (9oz) shelled fresh peas or frozen peas (or petits pois)
4 Little Gem lettuces, quartered
8 sprigs mint, shredded
Salt and freshly ground black pepper
pappardelle, cooked according to pack instructions, to serve
Olive oil and white wine vinegar, to serve (optional)

1. Preheat the oven to 150°C, 300°F, Gas 2. Season the meat. Heat the vegetable oil in a large, heavy, lidded casserole. Add the meat to the hot oil and brown on all sides. Remove it from the pan, cover and set aside, then brown the vegetables and garlic. Reduce the heat, add the butter and herbs, and mix well.

2. Add the tomato puree to the pan and sprinkle over the flour to coat the vegetables. Add the wine, lamb, bone and stock. Stir and bring gently to a simmer. Cover and cook in the centre of the oven for 1–1¼ hours or until tender. (You can prepare the dish up to this stage a day in advance – allow to cool and then refrigerate.)

3. Remove the meat from the gravy and set aside. Pass the gravy through a sieve – you want it to be slightly thick, not heavy or watery, so reduce over a low heat until you have the right consistency.

4. Return the gravy to the pan, along with the meat, and bring to a simmer over a medium heat. Reduce the heat, and add the peas and lettuce. Cover the pan and cook gently over a low heat for about 5 minutes, until the lettuce begins to wilt. Stir in the mint.

5. Toss the pasta with olive oil and white wine vinegar, if wished, and serve with the meat and vegetables.

POULTRY

ROASTED CHICKEN WITH CHEESE, ROASTED TOMATOES AND LEEKS

SERVES 2

1 leek, cut into 2.5 cm (1in) pieces
1 tbsp olive oil
salt and black pepper
2 chicken thigh and leg portions
75g (3oz) garlic and herb flavoured cream cheese (Philadelphia or Boursin)
3 medium tomatoes, halved
1 garlic clove, crushed
large pinch of caster sugar
4 sprigs fresh thyme

1. Preheat the oven to 190°C, 375°F, Gas 5. Place the leeks in a large roasting tin and drizzle with half the olive oil. Season with salt and black pepper. Roast for 15 minutes.

2. Meanwhile, carefully loosen the chicken skin with your fingers and rub the cream cheese between skin and flesh. Sit the chicken legs in the roasting tin on top of the leeks. Surround with the halved tomatoes.

3. Scatter the tomatoes with the garlic and a sprinkle of sugar (to bring out their natural sweetness). Tear the thyme sprigs over the chicken and season the whole dish with salt and pepper.

4. Drizzle with the remaining olive oil and roast for 45 minutes, or until the chicken is cooked. Pierce the flesh with a knife; if the juices run clear the chicken is ready.

5. Remove the chicken from the oven and rest for 5 minutes. Serve topped with the delicious sauce created by the melted cheese.

SPICED ROAST DUCK WITH CRANBERRY AND FIGS

SERVES 4

1 whole duck, weighing about 2.5kg (5½ lb)
salt and freshly ground black pepper
10 whole cloves
1 orange, halved
2 cinnamon sticks, bruised
150ml (¼ pt) red wine
½ x cranberry and fig relish

1. Preheat the oven to 200°C, 400°F, Gas 6. Remove the giblets from duck, rinse the duck inside and out, and pat dry. Lightly prick the skin all over with a fork, then season the duck inside and out with salt and pepper.

2. Stud cloves into the skin of the orange halves, then put them into the duck's body cavity with the cinnamon sticks.

3. Place the duck in a roasting tin. Roast for 20 minutes. Baste the duck with any melted fat, then turn the oven down to 180°C, 350°F, Gas 4. Cook for another 1 hour 10 minutes, or until the juices run clear when the thickest part of the leg is pierced.

4. Tip the fat out of the duck, then transfer to a serving platter.

5. Discard the fat in the roasting tin. Place the tin over a medium heat. Pour in red wine, loosening sediment with a wooden spoon. Stir in relish. Cook, stirring, for 2 minutes. Pour some sauce over the duck, and serve with the remainder on the side.

VEGETABLE AND CHICKEN SKEWERS

SERVES 4

1 red pepper
1 yellow pepper
1 small courgette
1 red onion

5 cherry tomatoes
2 skinned chicken breasts, cooked
1 bag mixed salad leaves
4 tablespoons low-fat salad dressing

1. Cut the vegetables and the cooked chicken roughly into 2.5cm (1in) pieces and thread onto skewers.
2. Place the skewers onto a hot barbecue and leave until the vegetables start to brown at the edges, turning halfway through.
3. When cooked, place the kebabs onto a plate of salad leaves and drizzle with the salad dressing.

JERK CHICKEN BURGERS

SERVES 4

For the marinade:
2 tbsp vegetable oil
1 small onion, sliced
2 garlic cloves, crushed
2 tbsp Dunn's River jerk seasoning
zest and juice of 1 lime

For the burger:
4 skinned chicken breasts
salt
4 wholegrain rolls
olive oil
4 tbsp mayonnaise
a few lettuce leaves
2 medium tomatoes, sliced

1. Mix all the ingredients for the marinade and rub onto the chicken. Marinate for at least 30 minutes or leave overnight in the fridge.
2. Season chicken with salt and barbecue or grill over a medium heat, turning now and then, for 18–20 minutes until cooked through.
3. Cut the rolls open and brush with olive oil. Lay cut side down on the barbecue to grill for 1 minute. Sandwich the mayo, lettuce, tomatoes and chicken into the roll and serve.

RED CHICKEN WITH CUBAN RICE ⭐

SERVES 4

1 tbsp olive oil
1 tbsp vegetable oil
juice of 1 lime
½tsp cayenne pepper
½tsp paprika
4 skinless and boneless chicken breasts
1 onion, finely chopped
1 green pepper, deseeded and finely chopped
250g (9oz) easy-cook long-grain rice
350ml (12fl oz) water or chicken stock (made with ½ cube)
handful chopped parsley
handful chopped coriander
lime wedges to garnish

1. Mix together the olive oil, lime juice, cayenne pepper and paprika and marinate the chicken breasts.
2. Heat the vegetable oil in a saucepan and sauté the onion and green pepper. Add the rice and mix well, then stir in the water or chicken stock and simmer for 10 minutes or until the rice is cooked.
3. Meanwhile, cook the chicken in a non-stick frying pan or on a ridged grill pan for 15–20 minutes until cooked through.
4. Add the parsley and coriander to the rice and serve with the chicken and lime wedges to squeeze over.

CHICKEN BREASTS WITH BACON AND PEAS

SERVES 2

1 tbsp vegetable oil
15g (½oz) butter
2 chicken breast fillets
1 small onion
4 rashers *Finest* streaky bacon, chopped
150ml (¼pint) *Finest* fresh chicken stock
juice of ½ an orange
100g (3½oz) shelled fresh or frozen peas

1. Heat the vegetable oil and the butter in a non-stick frying pan. Season the chicken fillets and brown for 5–7 minutes each side. Remove from the pan and slice into strips.
2. Add the onion to the pan along with the streaky bacon. Cook until golden then add the chicken stock, orange juice and peas. Bring to a simmer, return the chicken strips to the pan and simmer, covered, for 2–3 minutes.
3. Serve with new potatoes.

SPICY CHICKEN PIECES TANDOORI-STYLE

SERVES 6

1 x 500g tub natural yogurt
3 garlic cloves, crushed
2.5cm (1in) freshly grated ginger
2 tsp paprika
1 tsp ground cumin
1 tsp ground coriander
1 ½ tsp ground cinnamon
¼ tsp ground cloves
2 tsp salt and freshly ground black pepper
1.5kg (3lb 5oz) chicken pieces, skin on

1. In a large bowl mix the natural yogurt with the garlic, ginger, paprika, cumin, coriander, cinnamon and cloves. Season to taste with salt and pepper.

2. Take the chicken pieces and, with a sharp knife, make 2–3 deep cuts in each. Add the chicken to the yogurt marinade and work the mixture well into the cuts. Cover and leave to marinate in the fridge for 8 hours.

3. Lightly brush the barbecue or grill with oil. Scrape the excess marinade from the chicken pieces, then barbecue or grill them over a medium heat for 30–40 minutes, turning once, until tender and cooked through.

4. Serve immediately with lime wedges and naan bread.

CAESAR SALAD WITH WARM CHICKEN AND ASPARAGUS ✪

SERVES 4

4 tbsp vegetable oil
2 thick slices wholegrain bread from a small loaf (about 40g/1½oz each), crusts removed and diced
2 tbsp olive oil
4 skinned chicken breast fillets, seasoned
1 x 250g pack asparagus, trimmed and halved lengthways
1 x pack romaine lettuce hearts, torn in large bite-sized pieces
1 x pack fresh chives, cut in short lengths
6–8 tbsp Caesar dressing
50g (1¾oz) freshly shaved Parmesan
salt and freshly ground black pepper

1. Heat the vegetable oil in a large non-stick frying pan and fry the cubes of bread over a medium heat until crisp and golden to make croutons. Drain on kitchen paper.

2. Heat the olive oil and cook the chicken over a medium heat for 15–20 minutes until cooked through. Leave to rest for 5 minutes, then cut into slices. Saute the asparagus in the same pan until tender.

3. Toss the lettuce and chives with the dressing. Arrange on four plates and top with the chicken, asparagus, croutons and Parmesan. Season and serve at once.

LEMON CHICKEN, ROCKET AND PASTA SALAD

SERVES 6

3 lemons, thinly sliced
4 boneless, skinless chicken breasts
300g (10½oz) dried fusilli (or any other short shaped pasta you prefer)
2 x 50g pack Tesco *Finest* Wild Rocket Salad
50g (1¾ oz) pine nuts, lightly toasted
50g (1¾oz) Parmesan, finely grated
salt and freshly ground black pepper

For the dressing:
5 tbsp mayonnaise
5 tbsp milk
1 garlic clove, crushed
3 tbsp chopped fresh tarragon
finely grated zest and juice of ½ lemon
1 tsp clear honey
1 tsp Dijon mustard
salt and freshly ground black pepper

1. Line a bamboo steamer with half the lemon slices. Place the chicken on top of the slices, season and cover with the remaining lemon slices. Cover the steamer and place it over a saucepan of boiling water and steam for 12–15 minutes or until the chicken is cooked through. Discard the lemon slices and set the chicken aside to cool.

2. Cook the pasta according to the pack instructions, drain and set aside to cool.

3. Make the dressing by whisking together all the dressing ingredients in a bowl until smooth. Season.

4. To assemble the salad, slice the cooled chicken and place it in a large bowl with the cooked pasta. Add the rocket and stir in the dressing to coat. Sprinkle over the pine nuts and Parmesan and serve at room temperature.

CHICKEN BURGERS WITH BLUE CHEESE MAYONNAISE

SERVES 4

150ml (¼pt) mayonnaise
75g (3oz) blue cheese, crumbled
1 tbsp freshly chopped chives
500g (1lb 2oz) skinless and boneless chicken thighs
6 streaky bacon rashers
1 tbsp olive oil
1 garlic clove, crushed
1 shallot, chopped
2 tbsp freshly chopped tarragon
50g (1¾oz) wholegrain breadcrumbs
salt and pepper
4 wholegrain rolls
salad leaves to garnish

1. Mix the mayonnaise with the blue cheese and chives, and refrigerate.
2. Cut the chicken thighs and 2 streaky bacon rashers into pieces, then blend in a food processor until coarsely chopped.
3. Heat the oil in a frying pan, add the garlic and shallot and cook for 1–2 minutes until softened. Cool and add to the chicken mixture, along with the tarragon and breadcrumbs. Season and mix well.
4. Divide into four and, working with floured hands, shape into burgers. Grill the remaining 4 streaky bacon rashers over a medium heat for 8–10 minutes until crisp, and barbecue or grill the burgers over a medium heat for about 15 minutes, turning once, until tender and cooked through.
5. Toast 4 wholegrain rolls on the barbecue or under the grill. Arrange salad leaves on one half of each bun. Top with a chicken burger, a spoonful of mayonnaise and a bacon rasher, and the other half of the bun.

TURKEY MILANESE

SERVES 4

75g (3oz) fresh wholegrain breadcrumbs
zest of 1 lemon, finely grated
4 tbsp chopped parsley
4 skinned turkey breast steaks
25g (1oz) flour
1 large egg, beaten
1 tbsp vegetable oil
15g (½oz) butter
lemon wedges to garnish
salt and pepper

1. Combine the breadcrumbs, lemon zest and parsley and season generously.
2. Dip the turkey steaks in the flour and shake off excess, then dip the steaks into the beaten egg and finally into the breadcrumbs to coat evenly.
3. Heat the vegetable oil and butter in a non-stick frying pan and cook two steaks over a medium–high heat for 2–3 minutes each side until crisp and golden. Keep warm while you cook the other two in the same way.
4. Serve with steamed broccoli florets and garnished with the lemon wedges.

SPICY CHICKEN IN YOGURT

SERVES 4

4 skinless, boneless chicken breast fillets
300ml (½pt) natural yogurt
1 tsp ground turmeric
1 tsp ground ginger
1 tsp mild chilli powder
1 tsp ground coriander
2 tbsp vegetable oil
2 large onions, chopped
50g (1¾oz) creamed coconut
1 x pack fresh coriander leaves, chopped

1. Cut the chicken breasts into bite-sized pieces. In a mixing bowl, combine the yogurt, dried spices and chicken pieces. Place in the fridge until you are ready to use.

2. Heat the oil in a large frying pan or wok (with a lid) and gently fry the onions until soft. Add the chicken, spice and yogurt mixture, bring to a simmer, cover and cook gently for about 40 minutes. (The mixture will separate.)

3. Crumble the creamed coconut into the pan and stir until dissolved. Add the chopped coriander leaves, stir, and serve immediately with organic brown rice, if wished.

CHICKEN IN GARLIC CREAM SAUCE WITH BROCCOLI FRITTERS

SERVES 6

1 small onion, finely chopped
15g (½oz) butter
1 tbsp vegetable oil
4 cloves garlic, crushed
1 x 284ml carton double cream
6 chicken breast fillets

For the fritters
500g (1lb 2oz) broccoli, finely chopped
225g (8oz) wholemeal flour
1 heaped tsp baking powder
2 eggs
175ml (6fl oz) milk
salt and freshly ground black pepper
vegetable oil for frying

1. For the fritters, blanch the broccoli in boiling salted water for 2 minutes, drain, refresh in cold water, drain and pat dry.

2. Mix the flour, baking powder, eggs, milk and seasoning. Add the broccoli. Heat the oil in a pan and drop in spoonfuls of batter and cook over a medium heat until crisp.

3. Soften the onion in a pan with the butter and oil. Add the garlic and cream, then the chicken. Season, cover and simmer for about 20 minutes or until cooked. Serve at once.

DUCK BREASTS WITH GINGER AND LIME

SERVES 4

4 duck breasts, skin on
5cm (2in) piece fresh root ginger, peeled and finely shredded
thinly pared zest of 1 lime, cut into fine shreds
1 garlic clove, crushed
juice of 1–2 limes
2–3 tbsp dark soy sauce
2 tsp clear honey
1 tsp coriander seeds, crushed
1 tbsp vegetable oil
1 small onion, finely chopped
1 x 300ml tub *Finest* fresh chicken stock
salt and freshly ground black pepper
lime wedges to garnish

1. With a sharp knife, score the skin of the duck breasts, making several parallel cuts, not too deep, about 5mm (¼in) apart. Season. Chop half the shredded ginger and lime zest and mix in the garlic, juice of 1 lime, 1 tbsp soy sauce, the honey and coriander seeds. Spread this over the non-skin side of the duck and marinate for at least 1 hour.

2. Preheat the oven to 200°C, 400°F, Gas 6. Scrape off the marinade and reserve. Heat a frying pan over a medium heat and add the duck, skin-side down. Cook for 5 minutes, until the skin is browned but not burnt. Place the duck skin-side up on a baking sheet, spread over the reserved marinade and cook in the oven for 12–15 minutes. Cover and keep warm.

3. Meanwhile, add the oil to the frying pan and cook the onion until softened. Add the remaining ginger and cook for 2–3 minutes. Add the stock and remaining lime zest and simmer until slightly reduced. Add the remaining soy sauce and simmer until slightly thickened. Add more lime juice, honey and seasoning to taste.

4. Serve the duck breasts, cut into slices, skin-side up with the sauce and garnished with lime wedges.

FISH

ROASTED COD WITH BACON, TOMATOES AND THYME
SERVES 6
2 x large cod fillets, each weighing approx 650g (1lb 7oz)
salt and freshly ground black pepper
6 bacon rashers
1 x 500g pack cherry tomatoes
8 sprigs of fresh thyme
2 tbsp olive oil

1. Preheat the oven to 200°C, 400°F, Gas 6. Line a large roasting tin with greaseproof paper. Sit the cod with the skin side down in the tin and season with salt and pepper.
2. Top the fillets with bacon and scatter with the tomatoes and thyme, then drizzle with olive oil. Roast for 15–18 minutes until the fish is cooked through and the bacon has turned crisp.

GRILLED SARDINES WITH CAPERS AND MINT
SERVES 4
8–12 very large or 16–24 medium-sized sardines
sea salt and freshly ground black pepper
75g (3oz) unsalted butter
6 tbsp capers, chopped
1 pack fresh mint, roughly chopped

1. The sardines should be scaled, the heads removed and gutted, then washed and dried. Preheat the grill to maximum. Make 2–3 cuts in each side of the sardines, then sprinkle with sea salt and pepper. Cook for 3–5 minutes each side until the skin is lightly charred and the flesh firm to the touch.
2. Meanwhile, melt the butter in a small pan until it turns golden. Stir in the capers and allow to soften for 1 minute, then stir in the fresh mint.
3. Pour over the sardines and serve at once with crusty bread and a tomato and onion salad.

TUNA SPAGHETTI WITH CHUNKY TOMATOES, LEMON AND BASIL

SERVES 4

350g (12oz) spaghetti
2 x 185g tin tuna
5 medium tomatoes, roughly chopped
4 tbsp olive oil
zest and juice of 1 lemon
1 garlic clove, crushed (optional)
salt and freshly ground black pepper
a handful of fresh basil leaves

1. Cook the pasta in a large pan of salted, boiling water, according to packet instructions, until 'al dente' (just tender to the bite), then drain.
2. Meanwhile, drain the tuna and toss in a large bowl with the tomatoes, olive oil, lemon zest and juice, and garlic (if using). Season generously with salt and freshly ground black pepper.
3. Add the drained pasta into the fresh tuna and tomato sauce. Tear the basil leaves, add to the bowl, give it all a gentle mix and serve immediately.

SALMON TERIYAKI WITH SESAME NOODLES

SERVES 4

4 salmon fillets, approx 175g (6oz)
½ tbsp chopped fresh ginger
1 garlic clove, crushed
3 tbsp Kikkoman teriyaki marinade
2 tbsp sesame seeds
1 tbsp vegetable oil
salt
1 x 200g pack Tesco Traditionally Sliced Runner Beans
noodles, to serve

1. Place the salmon in a shallow china or glass dish, rub with ginger, garlic and teriyaki, and cover. Marinate for 30 minutes or overnight in the fridge.

2. Heat a large heavy-based frying pan over a low heat. Add the sesame seeds and toast, stirring, until golden. Transfer to a bowl and return the pan to a medium heat. Pat the salmon dry and brush with the oil. Season with salt and cook, skin side up, for 4 minutes. Turn the fillets, cooking for 3 minutes for pink or 4 minutes if you prefer your salmon cooked through.

3. Meanwhile, cook the sliced runner beans in a saucepan of salted boiling water, for 3–4 minutes, until just tender, and drain thoroughly.

4. Place the fish on a bed of beans and scatter with the toasted sesame seeds. Serve with noodles.

LEEK AND SMOKED SALMON SUPPER

SERVES 4

60g (2¼oz) butter
1 large leek, sliced
350g (12oz) dried egg tagliatelle
150g smoked salmon trimmings,
cut into small pieces
1 x 200g tub low-fat crème fraiche
60g (2¼oz) Parmesan cheese, grated
freshly ground black pepper

1. Heat the butter in a large frying pan until melted, then add the leek and sauté over low heat until tender.

2. Meanwhile, cook the pasta according to pack instructions.

3. Add the salmon to the pan and gently heat through, then add the crème fraiche, stirring well to combine. Add some pepper and half of the Parmesan to the sauce and stir until heated through again. Drain the pasta and combine with the sauce. Serve with the remaining Parmesan and some black pepper on top.

PRAWN AND SQUID JAMBALAYA

SERVES 4

1 tbsp vegetable oil

1 onion, finely chopped

2 celery stick, thickly sliced

2 red peppers, deseeded and cut into 2.5cm (1in) squares

1 x 200g packet cubed bacon

½ tsp hot cayenne pepper

1 tsp dried oregano

½tsp dried thyme

300g (10½oz) brown rice

450ml (16fl oz) chicken stock

1x 400g tin chopped tomatoes

200g (8oz) squid, cut into rings

1x 200g pack Tesco Finest Cooked Freshwater Prawns

3 spring onions, thinly sliced

1. Heat the oil in a large heavy-based saucepan with a tight-fitting lid. Stir in the onion, celery, red peppers and bacon. Cover and cook over a low heat for 5 minutes to start softening. Stir in the cayenne pepper, oregano and thyme and cook for a further 2 minutes.

2. Now add the rice. Cook, stirring for 1 minute, then pour in the stock and the chopped tomatoes. Bring to the boil and cover. Reduce the heat and simmer gently for 30–35 minutes.

3. Using a fork, stir in the squid, prawns and spring onions. Remove from the heat, cover and leave to stand for 5 minutes, until the squid is cooked and the rice is nice and fluffy.

SPICE-CRUSTED TUNA WITH CHERRY TOMATO COMPOTE ⭐

SERVES 4

2 tbsp coriander seeds
1 tbsp peppercorns
pinch of salt
4 tuna steaks (125–150g/4½–5½oz each)
2 tbsp olive oil
1 red pepper, deseeded and finely chopped
1 yellow pepper, deseeded and finely chopped
1 garlic clove, crushed
1 x 250g pack cherry tomatoes, halved
1 tsp wine vinegar
2 tbsp parsley, chopped

1. Roughly crush the coriander seeds and peppercorns with a pinch of salt and use to coat the tuna steaks.

2. Heat 1 tbsp of olive oil in a frying pan and quickly sauté the peppers. Add the garlic and cherry tomatoes, and turn in the pan for 1–2 minutes until just slightly softening. Remove from the heat and stir in the wine vinegar and parsley.

3. Put the rest of the olive oil in a non-stick frying pan or on a ridged grill pan and set over a high heat. Cook the tuna steaks for 2–4 minutes each side, depending on how well done you like them.

4. Serve with the compote, new potatoes and a green vegetable.

SEAFOOD CHOWDER ⭐

SERVES 4

2 tbsp vegetable oil
1 onion, chopped
2 celery sticks, chopped
3 new potatoes, unpeeled and diced
2 leeks, sliced
1 x 400g chopped tomatoes
1 x 300ml carton fish stock
300ml (½pt) water
1 bay leaf
a few sprigs of fresh thyme
2–3 strips orange zest
1 x 400g pack seafood selection
freshly ground black pepper
freshly chopped parsley to garnish

1. Heat the vegetable oil and fry the onion and celery until softened. Add the potato, leeks, chopped tomatoes, fish stock, water, 1 bay leaf, a few sprigs fresh thyme and orange zest. Bring to a simmer, then cover and cook for 20 minutes.
2. Stir in the seafood selection and simmer for 10 minutes. Add pepper to taste. Garnish with parsley and serve with crusty wholegrain bread.

STUFFED TROUT ⭐

SERVES 6

6 trout, weighing about 250g (9oz) each
2 medium onions, thinly sliced
2 medium tomatoes, thinly sliced
75g (3oz) mushrooms, thinly sliced
1 tsp mixed herbs
1 tsp garlic powder
salt and freshly ground black pepper

1. Preheat the oven to 200°C, 400°F, Gas 6.
2. Wash the trout under cool running water and pat dry using kitchen paper. Fillet the fish (or ask the fish counter to do this for you).
3. Place six pieces of foil on a baking tray and lay one of the fillets on each.
4. Layer the onions, tomatoes and mushrooms on top of the fish fillets. Season the fillets and sprinkle with the mixed herbs and garlic powder. Lay the second fillets on top of the vegetables and bring the foil up around each fish to make a sealed package.
5. Cook in the centre of the oven for about 40 minutes. Open the foil packets at the table (the presentation is impressive) and serve with buttered jacket potatoes, sweetcorn or garden peas.

MUSSELS WITH GARLIC, TOMATO AND FRESH HERBS

SERVES 4
2 tbsp olive oil
1 onion, chopped
1kg bag mussels
1 x 250g pack cherry tomatoes, halved
2 garlic cloves, crushed
2 sprigs lemon thyme
150ml (¼pt) dry white wine
salt and freshly ground black pepper
2 tbsp flat leaf parsley, chopped

1. Heat the olive oil in a pan with a lid. Add the onion and cook, covered, for 5 minutes. Meanwhile, scrub the mussels under running water, pulling off the beards. Discard cracked or open ones that don't close when tapped.
2. Stir the tomatoes, garlic and lemon thyme into the pan; cook for 3 minutes. Pour in the wine, bring to the boil and season. After 2 minutes, add mussels. Cover and simmer for 3–4 minutes until the mussels have opened; discard any closed ones.
3. Sprinkle with the parsley and serve.

SCALLOP AND SALMON SKEWERS WITH HERBED POTATO SALAD

SERVES 4

For the green olive oil:
4 tbsp olive oil
1 tsp each chopped chives,
parsley and basil

For the balsamic reduction:
100ml (4fl oz) balsamic vinegar

For the skewers:
2 packs fresh rosemary
8 large king scallops
200–250g (7–9oz) piece thick salmon fillet,
skinned and cut into 8 even-sized pieces
1 tbsp olive oil
salt and freshly ground black pepper

For the salad:
400g (14oz) new potatoes,
such as Charlotte, scrubbed
125g (4½oz) fine green beans
3 tbsp olive oil
4 tbsp balsamic vinegar
25g (1oz) red onion, very finely sliced
2 small spring onions, very finely chopped
4 tsp chopped chives

1. To make the green olive oil, whizz the oil and herbs in a food processor. Season, strain through a sieve and store in the fridge.
2. To make the balsamic reduction, boil the vinegar in a saucepan and reduce by half. Cool, then store in the fridge.
3. Choose the eight best and most even-sized sprigs of rosemary from the

packs. Remove the rosemary spikes apart from those at the top of the sprigs and thread the fish onto them. Season and set aside.

4. Cook the potatoes in boiling salted water until just tender. Drain and peel and slice them, then set aside. Cook the beans in boiling salted water for about 3 minutes – they should stay bright green and crisp.

5. When almost ready to serve, heat 1 tbsp olive oil in a frying pan over medium heat and cook the skewers for about 2 minutes each side until cooked through. Warm the potatoes in 3 tbsp olive oil, then add the vinegar and remaining ingredients.

6. Divide the potato salad between the plates and top each with two skewers. Drizzle with the green olive oil and balsamic reduction round the plates and serve immediately.

TIGER PRAWN SALAD WITH LIME AND CORIANDER

SERVES 2

1 x 125g pack Tesco *Finest* New World Salad
2 tsp groundnut oil
2 tsp sesame oil
1 red pepper, deseeded and chopped
200g (7oz) cooked and peeled tiger prawns
juice of 1 lime
2 tbsp freshly chopped coriander
salt and freshly ground black pepper
a few sprigs of coriander to garnish

1. Place the salad in a serving bowl.

2. Heat the oils in a frying pan, add the pepper and prawns and sauté for 2–3 minutes. Transfer to a bowl and add the lime juice and coriander. Season, stir well and leave to cool.

3. Place the prawns and dressing over the salad and serve garnished with a few sprigs of coriander.

FISH KEBABS WITH AVOCADO SALSA

SERVES 4

600g (1lb 5oz) firm fish, such as monkfish and tuna
1 tsp ground coriander
1 tsp salt
1 tsp turmeric
½ tsp chilli powder
½ tsp ground cumin
1 tbsp tomato puree
2 tbsp vegetable oil
juice of 1 lime

for the salsa:
2 medium avocados, chopped
1 small red onion, chopped
2 tbsp chopped fresh coriander, chopped
1 tbsp lime juice
seasoning

1. Cut the fish into large cubes. Mix the ground coriander, salt, turmeric, chilli powder, ground cumin, tomato puree, vegetable oil and lime juice. Toss the fish to coat, cover and leave to marinade for at least 30 minutes.
2. Thread the fish onto four large or eight small skewers and cook under a preheated grill, basting occasionally, for about 10 minutes.
3. Make the salsa by combining all the ingredients. Serve with the kebabs and with warm flat bread or boiled rice.

VEGETARIAN

MUSTARDY POTATOES WITH GREEN BEANS AND LEMON DRESSING ⭐

SERVES 6

900g (2lb) new potatoes, peeled and
cut into 5cm (2in) chunks
250g (9oz) thick green beans, trimmed
3 tbsp olive oil
juice of 1 lemon
1 tsp whole-grain mustard
salt and black pepper

1. Place the potatoes in a large pan of cold water. Cover and bring to the boil. Turn down the heat and simmer for 15 minutes until almost tender. Add the beans and cook for 4 minutes further, until both are tender. Drain, saving some water for the pork gravy, and transfer to a serving dish.

2. Place the remaining dressing ingredients in a serving bowl, whisk, then toss the drained potatoes and beans in the dressing. Season with salt and pepper and serve.

SWEETCORN AND POTATO SOUP ⭐

SERVES 4

25g (1oz) butter
1 leek, finely sliced
4 new potatoes, unpeeled and cut into 1cm (½in) cubes
450g (1lb) frozen sweetcorn
a large pinch of ground nutmeg
850ml (1½pt) vegetable stock
100ml (3½fl oz) single cream or reduced-fat crème fraiche
1 tbsp snipped fresh chives
salt and freshly ground black pepper

1. Melt the butter in a large saucepan and stir in the leek. Cover and cook over a low heat for 5 minutes until the leek has softened, but not coloured.
2. Stir in the potatoes, sweetcorn, nutmeg and stock, and bring to the boil. Simmer for 10–12 minutes until the potatoes are cooked.
3. Whizz half the soup in a blender or food processor and return to the pan. Stir in the cream or crème fraiche, and warm through for 1 minute, without letting the soup boil. Stir in the chives, check the seasoning, and add salt and freshly ground pepper to taste.

STUFFED PEPPERS WITH TOMATOES, RED ONIONS AND CHEESE ⭐

SERVES 4

1 red onion, cut into wedges
1 tsp dried oregano
salt and freshly ground black pepper
3 tbsp olive oil
4 red peppers, halved lengthways and deseeded
3 medium tomatoes, quartered
150g (5½oz) mozzarella, sliced
1 tbsp fresh flat leaf parsley, roughly chopped

1. 1. Preheat oven to 220°C, 425°, Gas 7. Put the red onion wedges and oregano together into a bowl, season with salt and pepper, then stir in half the olive oil.

2. Drizzle the remaining olive oil into a roasting tin. Sit the halved peppers in the tin and stuff them with the prepared onions. Roast for 20 minutes until tender, then tuck the tomatoes around the onions. Top with the mozzarella and roast for a further 6–8 minutes, until the cheese is bubbling and golden. Serve with a generous sprinkling of parsley.

VEGGIE CHILLI

SERVES 4

1 tbsp olive oil
1 onion, finely chopped
2 garlic cloves, chopped
2 tsp paprika or chilli powder
1 tsp ground cumin
2 x 420g tins kidney beans,
drained and rinsed
1 x 400g tin chopped tomatoes
1 or 2 squares of dark chocolate
salt
2 tbsp chopped fresh coriander
chopped fresh tomato , sour cream and rice to serve

1. Heat oil in a large saucepan over a medium heat. Cook onions for 5 minutes until beginning to soften. Stir in the garlic and spices, cooking for a further minute.

2. Add the beans, tinned tomatoes and chocolate. Season with salt and increase the heat to bring to the boil. Simmer for 20 minutes adding a little water if the chilli dries out too much.

3. Stir in the coriander and serve with a dollop of sour cream, chopped tomatoes and some plain rice.

BROCCOLI WITH A GARLIC AND LEMON DRESSING

SERVES 6

700g (1lb 9oz) broccoli
salt
juice and zest of 1 lemon
1 garlic clove, crushed
1 tbsp olive oil
freshly ground black pepper

1. Cut the broccoli into small florets and cook in a pan of boiling salted water for 3–4 minutes or until just tender. Drain and tip into serving bowl.
2. Meanwhile, whisk together the remaining ingredients and season with salt and pepper.
3. Toss the dressing into the drained broccoli and serve.

LEMON AND COURGETTE RISOTTO

SERVES 4

700ml (1¼pt) vegetable stock
75g (3oz) butter
1 onion, finely chopped
1 garlic clove, finely chopped
225g (8oz) risotto rice
150ml (5fl oz) dry white wine
2 large courgettes
zest of 1 lemon
juice of ½ lemon
2 tbsp grated Parmesan, plus shavings to serve

1. Bring the stock to the boil in a saucepan, then lower the heat to a slow simmer. Melt half the butter in a large, heavy-based saucepan over a low heat and gently cool the onion for 5 minutes, until softened. Add the garlic and rice; cook, stirring continuously, for 1 minute to coat in the butter and toast slightly. Pour in the wine and cook, stirring, until all the liquid has been absorbed.

2. Stir in one ladleful of simmering stock and adjust the heat – the rice should be at a slow simmer. Stir continuously until the stock has been absorbed and the rice parts when a wooden spoon is run through it. Then add another ladleful of stock and continue cooking in this way, adding stock and stirring as you go.

3. When the rice is almost tender to the bite, grate one courgette into the pan and add a final ladleful of stock. Cook, still stirring, for 1 more minute. Meanwhile, slice the remaining courgette and blanch in a pan of salted boiling water, for 2 minutes, until just tender. Drain and set aside.

4. Remove the rice from the heat and stir in the lemon zest and juice, grated Parmesan and remaining butter. Stir vigorously, until the butter has melted, then cover with a tight fitting lid and leave to stand for 1 minute. Serve the risotto on a bed of blanched courgettes, with a scattering of Parmesan shavings.

GRILLED TORTILLA CRISPS WITH YOGURT, CUCUMBER AND LEMON SALSA

SERVES 4
4 flour tortillas
2 tbsp olive oil
salt
¼ cucumber
1 x 200g tub Greek yogurt
zest and juice of ½ lemon
black pepper

1. Preheat the grill. Cut the tortillas into quarters and place on a baking sheet. Brush with a little olive oil and season with salt. Grill for 2 minutes on each side until crisp then transfer to a wire rack to cool.

2. For the salsa, cut the cucumber in half lengthways and, with a teaspoon, scoop out any seeds; discard. Thinly slice the cucumber, place in a bowl and fold in the yogurt, remaining olive oil, lemon zest and juice, and season with salt and freshly ground black pepper.

CHEESY MUSHROOMS

SERVES 4

8 large flat mushrooms
1 garlic clove, crushed
4 sprigs fresh lemon thyme or a large pinch of dried thyme
1 tbsp olive oil
salt and freshly ground black pepper
100g (3½oz) cheddar cheese, grated
green salad to serve

1. Place the mushrooms on a roasting sheet and scatter with garlic and thyme. Drizzle with the oil and season with salt and freshly ground black pepper.
2. Grill for 5 minutes, top with grated cheese and grill for 1 minute, until melted. Serve with a green salad.

COURGETTE FRITTATA

SERVES 4

2 tbsp olive oil
2 courgettes, thinly slice
2 garlic cloves, crushed
salt and black pepper
8 eggs
½ x 20g packet fresh chives, snipped
2 tbsp grated cheese (Parmesan, Cheddar or mozzarella)

1. Preheat the grill. Heat the oil in a 20cm (8in) ovenproof frying pan over a high heat. Add the courgettes and garlic, and season with salt and freshly ground black pepper. Cook, stirring regularly for 3 minutes.
2. Meanwhile, crack the eggs into a large bowl and stir in the chives and grated cheese. Season with salt and black pepper and beat lightly with a fork. Add the cooked courgettes and stir well to combine.
3. Tip the frittata mixture back into the frying pan and cook on a low to medium heat for 4 minutes, until the base is set and beginning to colour. Transfer to the grill for 4–5 minutes until just set and golden.

BUTTER BEAN, BABY SPINACH AND MOZZARELLA SALAD ⭐

SERVES 4

200g (7oz) butter beans
1 x 150g pack mozzarella, sliced
75g (3oz) baby spinach
½ tbsp honey
2 tbsp olive oil
salt and black pepper

1. Cook the butter beans in salted boiling water until tender, then drain and refresh in cold water.
2. Toss the beans, mozzarella and baby spinach together in a bowl.
3. To make the dressing, whisk together the honey and olive oil and season with salt and freshly ground black pepper. Dress the salad and serve.

CORN WITH LIME AND CHILLI BUTTER ⭐

SERVES 4

75g (3oz) butter
1 red chilli, deseeded and finely chopped
zest of 2 limes
4 corn cobs with husks

1. Melt butter over a low heat. Stir in chilli and lime zest, then remove from heat and leave to infuse for 15 minutes. Chill, then shape into a log and wrap in foil. Keep in the fridge.
2. Meanwhile, peel back husks and remove corn silk. Fold husks back over the corn, tie with string. Soak in cold water for an hour to prevent husks catching fire.
3. Cook over medium coals for 15 minutes, turning frequently. Remove husks and cook for 10 minutes, turning until kernels are slightly charred. Serve with a slice of the chilli butter.

COURGETTE, AUBERGINE, MINT AND FETA SALAD ⭐

SERVES 4

1 large aubergine, sliced thinly lengthwise
3 courgettes, sliced thinly lengthwise
4 tbsp olive oil
2 garlic cloves, crushed
½ x pack fresh mint, roughly chopped
salt and black pepper
100g (3½oz) feta cheese

1. Barbecue or grill all of the sliced vegetables over a medium heat for 8–10 minutes, turning halfway through the cooking. You might find that you have to do this in batches.
2. Meanwhile, place the olive oil, garlic and mint in a large bowl and season with plenty of salt and freshly ground black pepper.
3. As you remove the vegetables from the grill, place them immediately in the flavoured oil to cool. Stir the vegetables occasionally to combine the flavours thoroughly.
4. Just before serving, transfer the salad to a large serving platter and roughly crumble over the feta cheese.

VEGETABLE KORMA ⭐

SERVES 4

2 tbsp vegetable oil
1 red onion, cut into wedges
2 carrots, peeled and thickly sliced
1 cauliflower, broken into florets
1 green chilli, deseeded and chopped
2 garlic cloves, crushed
1 tbsp grated ginger
1 tsp ground cumin
¼ tsp ground coriander
1 tsp garam masala
1 tsp salt

150ml (5fl oz) vegetable stock
100g (3½oz) frozen peas
6 tbsp full-fat natural yoghurt

1. Heat the oil in a frying pan over a medium heat and add the onion. Cook for 3–4 minutes, until beginning to soften.

2. Add the carrots, cauliflower, chilli, garlic, ginger and spices, and cook for 3 minutes further. Pour in the stock, cover and cook for 6–7 minutes until almost tender.

3. Add the peas and cook for a further 2–3 minutes until all the vegetables are tender. Take off the heat and stir in the yoghurt until it has thickened.

PEA, TOMATO AND CROUTON SALAD

SERVES 6
200g (7oz) granary bread, cut into 2cm (¾in) chunks
4 tbsp (60ml) olive oil
salt and black pepper
5 medium tomatoes, cut into large chunks
1 garlic clove, crushed
1 tsp dried mint
500g (1lb 2oz) frozen peas

1. Preheat oven to 190°C 375°F, Gas 5. First, make the croutons. Place the chunks of bread on a baking sheet and toss with half the olive oil. Bake for 15 minutes until golden. Season with salt.

2. While the croutons are in the oven, mix the tomatoes, garlic and dried mint and the remaining olive oil in a bowl, season to taste with salt and black pepper and set aside.

3. Next, cook the peas in boiling water for 3 minutes or until they're tender, then drain them well and toss them with the tomatoes. Stir in the croutons into the salad just before serving.

ROASTED VEGETABLE WEDGES WITH GARLIC MAYONNAISE

SERVES 6

3 large carrots, peeled and sliced diagonally 2cm (¾in) thick
2 sweet potatoes, peeled and cut into wedges
450g (1lb) swede, peeled and cut into wedges
2 tbsp olive oil
1 tsp chilli flakes
1 tsp dried rosemary
salt
2 whole heads of garlic, sliced horizontally in half
100g (3½oz) mayonnaise

1. Preheat the oven to 190°C, 375°F, Gas 5. Place the vegetables in a large roasting tray and toss with the oil, chilli, rosemary and salt. Wrap the garlic in kitchen foil and add to the tray. Roast them for 45 minutes until the vegetables are lightly charred.
2. Remove the garlic from the oven 10 minutes early to make the garlic mayonnaise. Squeeze out as much of the pulp as you can, mixing it into a bowl with the mayonnaise. Serve the roast vegetables on a large platter with cocktail sticks and the garlic dip.

10 GI Food Listings

In the following pages you will find lists of product ranges available in Tesco. The foods have been divided into three groups – high GI (red), medium GI (yellow) and low GI (green).

Important: For those of you who are concerned about your weight, you should only eat the green-light foods that are in bold. In addition there are certain green-light foods that are particularly high in calories where you should limit the quantity you eat. These are marked with an asterisk (*).

Some of the foods listed cannot be GI tested by standard methods as they contain no or virtually no carbohydrate. However, for the purpose of including a complete balance of foods, they have been included in the listings and are marked with a cross (†).

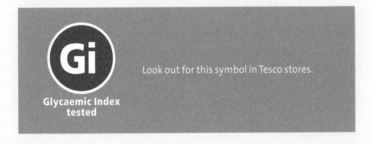

Gi

Glycaemic Index tested

Look out for this symbol in Tesco stores.

FRESH VEGETABLES †
Broad beans

FRESH VEGETABLES †

Alfalfa sprouts	Okra
Asparagus	Olives*
Aubergine	Onions
Beans	Parsley
(green/runner)	Peppers
Bok choy	Peppers (chillis)
Broccoli	Pickles
Brussels sprouts	Radicchio
Cabbage	Radishes
Capers	Sauerkraut
Carrots	Scallions
Cauliflower	Spinach
Celery	Sugarsnap peas
Collard Greens	Swiss Chard
Courgettes	Tomatoes
Cucumber	Yams
Garden peas	
Lettuce	
Mangetout	
Mushrooms	
Mustard greens	

FROZEN VEGETABLES †
Baby broad beans

FROZEN VEGETABLES †
Corn on the cob
Garden peas
Peas
Petits pois
Sweetcorn

FRUITS – FRESH
Cantaloupe
Honeydew Melon
Raisins
Watermelon

FRUITS – FRESH
Apricots
Bananas
Kiwi
Mangos
Papaya
Pineapple

FRUITS – FRESH

Apples	Mandarins
Cherries	Nectarines
Clementines	Oranges
Grapefruit	Peaches
Grapes	Pears
Lemons	Plums
Limes	Satsumas

BERRIES
Blackberries
Blueberries
Raspberries
Strawberries

OTHER
Avocado° (limit to 1/4)
Guavas
Plantain
Rhubarb

FRUITS – BOTTLED, TINNED, FROZEN, DRIED
Apple sauce (no sugar)
Frozen berries
Mandarin Oranges
Peaches in juice or water
Pears in juice or water

PASTA AND NOODLES (DRIED)
Capellini
Cellophane noodles (mung bean)
Cellentani pasta
Conchiglie pasta shells
Creste
Egg lasagne
Egg tagliatelle
Eliche pasta
Farfalle pasta
Fettuccine
Fusilli pasta twists
Lasagne
Lasagne sheets
Linguine
Lumache pasta
Macaroni
Noodles (frozen, express Chinese Oriental)
Penne
Radiatore
Rigatoni
Spaghetti
Tagliatelle
Vermicelli

FRUITS – BOTTLED, TINNED, FROZEN, DRIED
Apple puree containing sugar
Tinned Fruit in Syrup

PASTA
All tinned pasta
Gnocchi

Noodles (tinned)

STUFFINGS
Manor born sage & onion stuffing
Sage & onion stuffing mix
Tesco Finest herb stuffing mix
Tesco Finest pork, chestnut & onion stuffing
Tesco Finest pork, ham & leek stuffing
Tesco Finest pork, sage and onion stuffing

BAGELS
Original bagels
Plain bagels
Sundried tomato bagels
Tesco Finest bagels
Tesco Finest brunch bagels

FRUITS – BOTTLED, TINNED, FROZEN, DRIED
Dried Apples
Dried Cranberries
Extra fruit/low-sugar spreads
Fruit Cocktail in juice
Peaches/pears in syrup
Pineapple slices/chunks
Prunes
Sultanas

POTATOES
New potatoes
Sweet potatoes

BREADS

Bakers Premier Gold thick sliced white bread
Crispbreads
Croissants
Crusty white bloomer
Crusty white sliced
Doughnuts
French bread baguette
French bread cobs
French bread floured batard
French bread grand rustique
French bread ploughman's rolls
Hamburger buns
Healthy Living white loaf medium sliced
Homebake half baguettes
Homebake mini petit pains
Hot dog buns
Kaiser rolls
Mega Value 24 white rolls
Mini white pitta bread
Muffins
Organic white
Pancakes
Part-baked petits pains
Pikelets
Pizza
Premium white extra thick
Premium white medium
Round crusty rolls
Scottish plain white sliced
Single French country roll
Single white continental morning rolls

BREADS

10 Mini white pitta bread
Brown Multi Grain loaf
Crispbread with fibre
Finest multigrain batch bread
Finest oatmeal batch bread
Organic malt loaf
Sliced fruit loaf
Value white pitta bread
White Multi Grain loaf
Wholegrain breads
Wholemeal pitta bread

NUTS AND DRIED FRUIT

Dried, mixed fruit

FRESH PASTA (NOT FILLED)

Egg fusilli
Egg penne
Egg spaghetti
Egg spirals/fusilli
Egg tagliatelle

BREADS

100% stone-ground wholemeal
Crispbreads (high-fibre)
Finest crusty malted wheat loaf (800g)
Wholegrain, high-fibre breads

RICE

Indian Basmati rice
Indian Easy Cook Basmati rice
Organic Basmati rice
Value Basmati rice

NUTS AND DRIED FRUIT

Almonds* (see page 48)
Apricots
Cashew nuts*
Hazelnuts* (see page 48)
Macadamia nuts* (see page 48)
Mixed nuts & raisins*
Monkey nuts*
Pistachio nuts* (see page 48)
Prunes
Ready to eat pears
Roasted salted mixed*

BREADS CONT
Single white crusty round rolls
Stayfresh white medium
Stayfresh white thick
Tesco Finest country loaf
Tesco Finest crusty white
Tesco Finest French baguette
Tesco Finest French bread baton
Tesco Finest French bread ficelle
Tesco Finest French bread
Parisienne
Tesco Finest French bread petit
pains
Tesco Finest French cob
Tesco Finest French country loaf
Tesco Finest French Couronne
bread
Tesco Finest fruit & cinnamon
bread
Tesco Value white rolls
Tesco Value malt loaf
Tesco Value rolls, thick sliced
Tesco Value white medium sliced
Tesco Value white pitta bread
Tesco Value white thick sliced
Waffles
White Continental morning rolls
White Danish medium or thick
sliced
White loaf medium or thick
sliced
White sliced sandwich

CEREAL GRAINS
Amaranth
Croutons
Millet
Rice (short-grain, white, instant)
Rice cakes

CEREAL GRAINS
Barley
Buckwheat
Bulgar
Gram flour
Kasha (toasted buckwheat)
Soya Protein Powder
Wheat berries
Wheatgrain

BEANS & PULSES
Baked beans
Bartolli beans
Black eye beans
Butter beans
Cannellini beans
Chick peas
Chilli beans
Lageolet beans
Green lentils
Haricot/navy beans
Italian beans
Lentil dahl
Lima beans
Mixed beans Italienne
Mung beans
Peas
Pearl barley
Petits pois & Baby Carrots
Pinto beans
Pigeon peas
Red kidney beans
Red split lentils
Romano beans
Soy beans
Three bean salad
Yellow split peas
Baked beans
Baked beans in tomato sauce
Black eye beans
Butter beans
Cannellini beans

CEREALS
Cornflakes
Frosted flakes
Healthy Living muesli
Healthy Living Sultana Bran
Honey & Nut cornflakes
Tesco Value cornflakes
Tesco Value frosted flakes

MEAT, POULTRY, FISH, EGGS AND SOY †
Beefburgers
Hot dogs
Minced beef (more than 10% fat)
Pâté
Processed meats
Sausages
Sushi (rice based)
Whole regular eggs

CEREALS
Fruit muesli
Fruit & Fibre breakfast cereal
Fruit & Nut muesli
Tesco Value Fruit & Fibre
Tesco Value muesli
Wholewheat muesli

MEAT, POULTRY, FISH, EGGS AND SOY †
Chicken/turkey leg
Lamb (Tenderloin, Centre loin chop, Boiled ham)
Minced beef (lean)
Pork (Fore shank, Leg shank, Centre cut, Loin chop)
Sirloin tip
Sirloin steak
Turkey bacon
Whole omega-3 eggs

Chick peas
Green lentils
BEANS & PULSES (CONT)
Mixed salad beans
Petits pois & baby carrots
Red kidney beans
Red kidney beans – no added sugar or salt
Sweetcorn

CEREALS
**Healthy living branflakes
Hi fibre bran breakfast cereal
Oat Bran
Organic Porridge oats
Porridge oats
Scottish Porridge oats
Soya Protein Power
Tesco Value Porridge oats**

MEAT, POULTRY, FISH, EGGS AND SOY †
**All seafood, fresh, frozen or tinned (avoid breaded or battered)
Lean bacon°
Lean Beef
Chicken Breast (skinless)
Egg whites
Lean deli ham
Minced beef (extra lean)
Pork tenderloin
Quorn
Rabbit
Sashimi
Soy/whey powder
Tofu
Turkey breast (skinless)
Veal**

BISCUITS
50% reduced fat cream crackers
Cream crackers
Dutch crispbakes
Dutch melba toast
French toast
Nice biscuits
Original mini breadsticks
Rich tea biscuits
Rich tea finger biscuits
Tesco Value rich tea biscuits

DAIRY
Almond milk
Cheese
Cottage Cheese
Cream
Cream cheese
Evaporated milk
Rice milk
Sour cream

SOUPS
All cream-based soups
Pureed vegetable
Tinned black bean
Tinned green pea
Tinned split pea

BISCUITS
Digestive biscuits

DAIRY
Cheese (low-fat)
Cream cheese (light)
Crème fraiche (low-fat)
Frozen yoghurt (low-fat, low-sugar)
Ice-cream (low-fat)
Sour cream (light)

SOUPS
Tinned chicken noodle
Tinned lentil
Tinned tomato

TESCO READY MEALS *
Beef lasagne (frozen)
Beef stew with dumplings
Chicken chow mein
Chicken fajitas
Chicken tikka masala with rice
Chicken szechuan
Chilli beef
Cottage pie
Crispy aromatic duck
Crispy aromatic half chicken
Cumberland fish bake
Cumberland pie
Finest chicken korma & peshwari rice
Finest Chilli beef noodles
Finest Lasagne
Finest Tandoori chicken masala & rice
Finest Beef & ale casserole
Healthy Living chicken chow mein
Healthy Living chicken korma & rice
Healthy Living chicken tikka masala/rice
Healthy Living meat lasagne
Lasagne
Loaded potato skins
Mushroom burger
Mushroom stroganoff with rice
Roasted winter vegetables
Sausage & mash
Spinach & ricotta cannelloni
Shepherds pie
Finest lamb moussaka
Sweet and sour chicken
Sweet & sour chicken with noodles
Tomato & mozzarella bake
Value Cottage pie
Value Lasagne

YOGHURTS AND DESSERTS
Bourbon Vanilla yoghurt (Tesco Finest)*
Lemon Curd yoghurt (Tesco)

MILK AND PROBIOTICS
Cranberry (probiotic drink)
Pink grapefruit (probiotic drink)

COUSCOUS
Coriander & lemon couscous
Couscous
Mediterranean couscous
Wild mushroom couscous

FATS/OILS/DRESSINGS †
Corn oil
Mayonnaise (light)
100% Peanut butter
Peanut oil
Salad dressings (fat-free/low-sugar)
Sesame oil
Sunflower oil
Vegetable oils
Vinaigrette

FATS/OILS/DRESSINGS †
Butter
Coconut oil
Hard Margarine
Lard
Palm oil
Peanut butter
Salad dressings (regular)
Tropical oils
Vegetable Shortening

Vegetarian lasagne

YOGHURTS AND DESSERTS
Fruit yoghurts
Natural yoghurt (low-fat with sweetner)

MILK AND PROBIOTICS
British pasteurised semi-skimmed milk
British pasteurised skimmed milk
British pasteurised standardised homogenised milk
Fresh organic pasteurised whole milk *
Organic pasteurised semi-skimmed milk
Orange probiotic drink

OTHER DAIRY
Buttermilk
Cheese (fat-free)
Cottage Cheese (low-fat or fat-free)
Ice-cream (low-fat and no added sugar)
Sour cream (fat-free)
Soy cheese/low fat
Soya milk (plain/low-fat)

FATS/OILS/DRESSINGS †
Canola oil/rapeseed oil
Flax seed oil
Mayonnaise (low-fat/sugar)
Olive oil
Salad Dressings (low fat/sugar)
Soft margarine (non-hydrogenated, light)
Vegetable oil Sprays

SNACKS
Cereal/Granola bars
Chips
Chocolates
Crisps/Pretzels/Tortilla chips
Ice-cream (regular)
Jelly
Popcorn (regular)
Rice cakes
Sorbet

CONDIMENTS/SEASONINGS †
Ketchup
Mayonnaise
Tartar Sauce

SWEETS
Jelly babies

SUGAR AND SWEETENERS
Corn syrup
Glucose
Honey
Molasses
Sugar (all types)
Treacle

BEVERAGES
Active glucose drink
Active orange drink
Active sparkling orange drink
Active sport drink (lemon and orange)
Alcoholic drinks (In Phase II a glass of wine and the occasional beer may be included)
Fruit drinks

SNACKS
Dark chocolate (70% cocoa)
Popcorn (light, microwaveable)

SUGAR AND SWEETENERS
Fructose

BEVERAGES
Diet soft drinks (caffeinated)
Red wine (In Phase II)
Unsweetened fruit juices

SNACKS*
Food bars (20–30g carbs, 12-15g protein, 4-5g fat)
Tortillas

CONDIMENTS/SEASONINGS †
Chilli Powder
Extracts (Vanilla etc.)
Flavoured vinegars/sauces
Garlic
Herbs/Spices
Horseradish
Hummus*
Lemon/lime juice
Mustard
Peppers (all types)
Salsa (low-sugar)
Soy sauce (low-sodium)
Terriyaki sauce*
Worcestershire sauce

SUGAR AND SWEETENERS
Aspartame
Hermesetas Gold
Splenda
Stevia

BEVERAGES
Bottled water
Decaffeinated coffee
Diet soft drinks (no caffeine)
Herbal teas
Instant hot chocolate (light)
Soya milk (low fat, plain)

BEVERAGES (CONT)
Kick stimulation drink (all)
Prune juice
Regular coffee
Regular soft drinks
Sweetened juice
Watermelon juice

Tea (with skimmed milk)
Tonic water
FRUIT JUICES
Pure apple juice
Pure orange juice
Value apple juice
Value grapefruit juice
Value orange juice

TESCO LOW-GI RANGE
Tesco Low Gi Breakfast Bar –
Apple and Blackberry
Tesco Low Gi Breakfast Bar –
Almond and Redberry
Tesco Low Gi Ready to Drink –
Blackcurrant and Blueberry
Tesco Low Gi Ready to Drink –
Strawberry

TESCO WHOLEFOODS RANGE
Cous Cous
Udon Noodles

TESCO WHOLEFOODS RANGE
Apricots
Brazil nuts
Cashew nuts
Fruit & Nut Mix
Hazelnuts
Macadamia nuts
Mixed nuts
Monkey nuts
Pecan nuts
Pine nuts
Pistachio nuts
Prunes
Walnut halves
Whole almonds
Aduki beans
Black turtle beans
Butter beans
Cannellini beans
Chickpeas
Exotic bean mix
Haricot beans
Lentils
Mung beans
Pearl Barley
Red kidney beans
Soya beans
Bulgar wheat

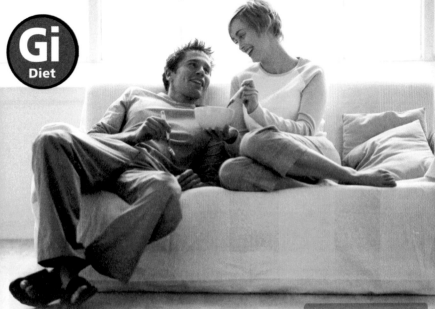

A personalised Gi diet to suit your lifestyle?

At Tesco Diets, we can provide you with a tailored Gi diet to suit the way you live your life, your health requirements, your food preferences and your weight loss objectives.

Click on **www.TescoDiets.com** and complete our FREE Diet profile. When you join we'll provide you with your first week's personalised meal plan and shopping list. Subscriptions cost just £2.99 per week*.

The Tesco Gi Diet is only available at Tesco Diets, the UK & Ireland's leading online diet destination.

*minimum 10 week initial subscription

What we offer...

1) Customised weekly meal plans & shopping lists
2) Personalised fitness plans & workouts
3) Ongoing support from a team of professionals
4) Confidential access to nutritional experts
5) Peer group support & encouragement, 24/7
6) A host of tools & tips to help you succeed
7) And now you can earn Clubcard points too!

TESCO

www.tesco-diets.com

The largest range of low and medium Gi products in the UK now at Tesco

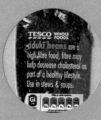

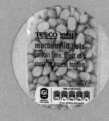

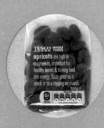

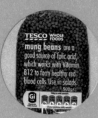

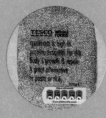

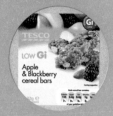

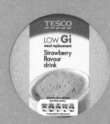

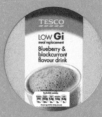

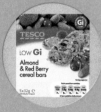

Please note that not all products will be available or labelled in all stores. Sign in at www.tesco.com and visit the Gi store in the grocery section to find out more.

TESCO | Every little helps

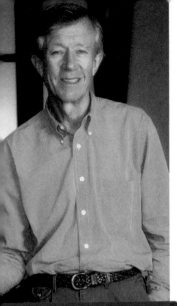

Formerly President of the Health & Stroke Foundation of Ontario for fifteen years, **Rick Gallop** is the author of the international bestseller *The Gi Diet*, *Living the Gi Diet*, *The Gi Diet Pocket Guide to Shopping & Eating Out* and most recently *The Family Gi Diet*. He lives in Toronto.

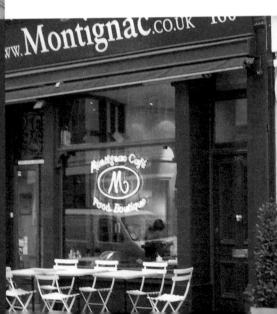

The Montignac Boutique and Café Since 1994
The original low Gi destination

160 Old Brompton Road
London SW5 0BA
Tel/Fax +44 (020) 7370 2010
www.montignac.co.uk
(See our website for mail-order)
mail@montignac.co.uk

Opening hours:
Monday - Fridays 8.30am-9.00pm
Saturday 8.30am-6.00pm
Sunday 10.00am-5.00pm

Special catering enquiries welcome
(Two days prior notice required -
thank you)

Also available from Rick Gallop and Virgin Books:

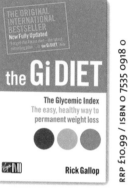

RRP £10.99 / ISBN 0 7535 0918 0

The original international bestseller – now fully revised and updated.

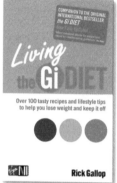

RRP £9.99 / ISBN 0 7535 0882 6

All the extra advice and support you need to stay motivated, along with 100 delicious recipes and new food lists so you can create your own meals.

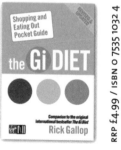

RRP £4.99 / ISBN 0 7535 1032 4

A pocket-sized reminder on which foods to buy at the supermarket, what to look for on labels and how to stay on track when eating out.

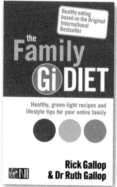

RRP £10.99 / ISBN 0 7535 1034 0

Healthy eating for the entire family – from little ones and fussy teenagers to mums-to-be and reluctant partners.

Index